LIFESTYLE AFTER COVID -19

BY

MUJAHID BAKHT

1

Hardcover: ISBN: 978-1-961299-48-1
Paperback: ISBN: 978-1-961299-49-8
EBook: ISBN: 978-1-961299-50-4
Audiobook: ISBN: 978-1-961299-59-7

Published by
Atlas Amazon, LLC
United States of America

Atlas Amazon, LLC.

244 Fifth Avenue, Suite D210

New York, NY 10001 USA

Hardcover: ISBN: 978-1-961299-48-1
Paperback: ISBN: 978-1-961299-49-8
EBook: ISBN: 978-1-961299-50-4
Audiobook: ISBN: 978-1-961299-59-7

Second Edition, August 2023

In "Lifestyle After COVID-19," acclaimed author Mujahid Bakht presents a timely and insightful exploration of the post-pandemic world and its profound impact on our well-being. Drawing upon the knowledge and experiences of the first edition, published in October 2022, this second edition delves even deeper into the challenges and opportunities that have emerged in the wake of the global COVID-19 crisis.

Mujahid Bakht guides readers through a comprehensive journey, addressing the physical, mental, and social dimensions of well-being in our rapidly evolving reality. With a compassionate and informed voice, the author unravels the complexities of our new normal and provides practical guidance on how to navigate the unique challenges we face.

From the importance of maintaining physical health through clean eating and physical exertion to nurturing robust mental health and forging meaningful social connections, "Lifestyle After COVID-19" offers invaluable insights for readers seeking to thrive in this transformed world. With a focus on resilience, adaptation, and holistic self-care, Bakht's book empowers individuals to embrace positive change and embark on a journey of personal growth and well-being.

Whether you are grappling with the long-term effects of the pandemic, seeking strategies to enhance your emotional resilience, or aiming to foster stronger social bonds, this second edition of "Lifestyle After COVID-19" is an indispensable guide, offering wisdom and practical tools to create a healthier and more fulfilling life in the midst of unprecedented global shifts.

TABLE OF CONTENTS

ACKNOWLEDGMENT

For my parents, my family, and my friends. Thank you for believing in me and trusting me. I dedicate this book to all of you who have encouraged me to become a better version of myself. Especially for my children, without whom it would have been impossible to accomplish this book.

You are all close to my heart

ABOUT AUTHOR

Mr. Mujahid Bakht, Profile:-

LIFE HISTORY:- Mr. Bakht is a mature, experienced, extremely enthusiastic, energetic, administrator and thirty-six years have proven experience as a businessman in international marketing and public relations. Mr. Bakht is an International Real Estate Specialist, and Professional Business and Projects Consultant. He was born in Pakistan, Educated in Pakistan and USA. Presently American Citizen belongs to the business-oriented family. Thirty-Seven years Resident of New York, USA.

BUSINESS HISTORY:- Mr. Bakht is a Founder & President of Atlas Amazon, LLC., Mr. Bakht is a business developer and multilingual business specialist in the Caribbean, South East Asia, and the Middle East emerging markets Mr. Bakht has served, met, and host many "Heads of the Countries" Also, maintain a close relationship with investors of high net worth in the USA.

CAREER:- Mr. Bakht has been engaged with many multinational companies in the field of international real estate investment, communication, technology, diamond, gold, mining, Pre-Feb housing, wind & solar energy, outsourcing management, and project consulting along with business partners & associates worldwide. Mr. Bakht has participated in major national and international conferences including participated in United Nations (U.N.O.) conferences.

TRAVEL:- Mr. Bakht is well-traveled and has visited many countries worldwide.

MANAGEMENT EXPERIENCE:- Thirty-Seven years of diversified experience in project consulting, marketing, and business management. As a Director of Marketing, Director of Public Relations, Director of International Affairs, Executive Vice President, President, CEO, and Chairman of many national & multinational companies, where he served previously. Mr. Bakht hired and trained many professionals as business consultants in international marketing and supervised them. Mr. Bakht is the author and publisher of multiple books.

CERTIFICATES; Certificate of Authenticity from Bill Rodham Clinton, President of the United States, and

Hillary Rodham Clinton First Lady, USA. (July 20, 2000);

CERTIFICATE OF ACHIEVEMENT; Achievement Award was presented to Mr. Bakht by Stephen Fossler for five years of continued growth and customer satisfaction from 1996 to 2001.

HONORS MEMBER; Madison Who's Who of Professionals, having demonstrated exemplary achievement and distinguished contributions to the business community, registered at the Library of Congress in Washington D.C. USA. (2007 & 2008)

HONORS MEMBER; Premiere Who's Who International, professional business executive having demonstrated exemplary achievement and distinguished contributions to the International business community, 2008 and 2009.

CERTIFICATE OF AUTHENTICITY; from Terence R. McAuliffe, Chairman of Democratic National Committee, Tom Dachle, Senate Democratic Leader, Dick Gephardt, House Democratic Leader, USA. (June 16, 2001);

CERTIFICATE OF AUTHENTICITY; from Terence R. McAuliffe, Chairman of Democratic National Committee, USA. (April 16, 2002).

PERSONAL HISTORY:- Mr. Bakht married in the year of 1992 in New York City, USA. He is a Father of three children, all three were Born raised, and educated in the United States of America.

Dartmouth College, New Hampshire, USA.
St. John University, Queens, New York, USA.
Syracuse University, Upstate New York, USA.

MEETINGS WITH DIGNITARIES AND HEADS OF THE COUNTRIES:

Honorable. Teng-Hui-Lee, President of Taiwan. 1999.
Hon. Leonard Fernandez, President of the Dominican Republic. 1999.
Prince. Ahmed Fahad Al-Turki, (Saudi Arabia). 2000.
Benazir Bhutto, Prime Minister of Pakistan, 2001.
Dr. Keith Mitchell, Prime Minister of Grenada, West Indies. 2003-2004.
Pierre Charles, Prime Minister of Dominica, West Indies,

2003.

Mr. Charles Sovran, Foreign Minister of Dominica, 2003.

Robert H. O. Corbin Leader & Deputy-Prime-Minister (PNC) Guyana 2004.

Hon. P. J. Peterson, Prime Minister of Jamaica. 2004.

Dr. Kenny D. Anthony, Prime Minister of Saint Lucia, West Indies. 2005.

Hon. Owen Arthur, Prime Minister of Barbados, West Indies. 2005.

Michael de la Bastide, "Chief Justice" and President of the Caribbean Islands. 2005.

Mahmood M. Hussain, the Private Office of His Royal Highness. Dr. Sheikh-

Sultan Bin Khalifa Bin Zayed Al Nahyan, Abu-Dhabi, U.A.E. 2005.

Sultan S. Al Mansoori, Saeed & Mohammed Alnaboodah, Dubai, UAE 2005.

Ibrahim A. Gambari, Under-Secretary-General (United Nations) 2006.

Hon. Villasarao Deshmukh, Chief Minister of Maharashtra, India, 2006.

Hon. Ashok Chovan, Minister of Industries, Maharashtra, India, 2006.

Hon. Liu Bowie, Ambassador of China, United Nations,

2006.

Senator Einstein Louison, Ministry of Agriculture, Grenada.

Hon. Mark Isaac, Minister of State, Grenada, West Indies.

Hon. Brenda Hood, Minister for Tourism, Civil Aviation, Culture, Grenada.

Wayne Smith, Mayor, Township of Irvington, New Jersey, USA.

Orlando J. Moreno, Brigadier General & Military Advisor, (UNO) Venezuela.

CHAPTER 1

INTRODUCTION

Despite being the most intellectual beings on planet, we humans fail to recognize the deeper, core purposes of life. How many times have you actually stopped and introspected? Introspection is ability very few of us have the privilege of practicing.

Is what you're doing in your career aligning with your goals? What happened to being an astronaut, a police officer when you were a child? In this race to achieve the most, we fail to achieve the valuable. There are many business tycoons struggling with their health despite all the money they could ask for.

The unease you feel in a job you don't like; the detachment you feel in a relationship you don't want to be in and the constant baggage you're carrying around is an indication. Your mind and body are screaming to you, calling out to you: Is your life a reflection of your well-being?

Have you ever asked yourself: who am I, and what am I capable of? Do you push your limits daily to achieve the maximum, from physical health, professional productivity relationships, happiness, and emotional capacity? Where do youstand in these areas of your life?

Well, these questions may feel uncomfortable to answer at this moment, but at the end of this book, you'll experience a journey you might've never been through. But before we get intothe specifics, let's delve into the term **well-being**. What does it mean?

What Is Well-being?

According to the Cambridge Dictionary, well-being is *the state of feeling healthy and happy.* Simple and easy right? Well, it may be true, but there's always more to the story. The term well-being is synonymous with positive mental health, a stable state of mind and body combined that allows you to grow and thrive. Well-being is defined as an experience of positive emotions and fulfillment, but it also reflects the growth of your potential, developing a sense of purpose in life, experiencing meaningful relationships, and last but not least, having control of your life.

It has been associated with professional, personal, and social improvement, with well-adjusted individuals exhibiting higher levels of workplace productivity, more learning motivation, cognitive flexibility, more prosocial behavior patterns, and positive relationships. However, well-being is a multi-faceted and contextual concept that follows no fixed formula. Many notable personalities have expounded upon well-being highlighting various aspects. The overall well-being is mainly defined by two theories which are proven or backed up by various other theories of philosophers and psychologists.

- **Hedonic well-being (HWB)**

Proposed by Diener in 1984, the HWB is a tripartite model that consists of

- Frequent pleasant feelings

- Infrequent unpleasant feelings

- Overall satisfaction from life

This theory talks about how satisfied one is with their life and if they are getting what they want. Because each person's pleasures are different this theory is also called subjective well-being and has a more selfish aspect. The 'things' in question that are pleasant or unpleasant to you may not only be different for another but are also irrespective of other people's desires and happiness.

- **Eudaimonic Well-being (EWB)**

EWB, in contrast to HWB, focuses on the psychological development and enhancement. This aspect of well-being revolves around the satisfaction one experiences by fulfilling their goals, moral obligations, needs and requirements. This means that the process to attain it may not always be easy or desirable. Also called psychological well-being, this theory is best drawn out by Ryff in 1989, building upon the concepts of Jung, Erikson, Rogers and Maslow.

These two theories have laid the foundation for many expertsto discuss, criticize and analyze the concepts of well-being in themost accurate and holistic manner.

Csikszentmihalyi theory about the state of flow in 1990 explained a person's level of engagement and concentration in relation with the difficulty or challenge of a situation. He stated that the flow state requires a very delicate balance between the difficulty level of the task and the skill set of the person doing it, where challenges should be a little more difficult than the skill set. This makes the task neither too difficult nor easy for the candidate. This is not necessarily followed by pleasure or happiness but the sense of fulfillment and achievement supports the EWB theory which talks about development and growth as well-being.

Some accounts of well-being (Boehm, Peterson, Kivimaki, & Kubzansky, 2011; Diener, Wirtz et al., 2010; Su, Tay, & Diener, 2014) include optimism which assumes that a person expects more positive experiences than negative ones in life. This theory helped experts positively relate optimism with better health status, lower levels of stress and depression and greater levels of happiness and satisfaction. Furthermore, Taylor and Brown were able to deduce that such 'positive illusion' about oneself, their future and the outcomes allows for functionality in adverse conditions. Therefore, it showed a strong correlation with EWB measures.

Perma theory by Dr. Seligman's, however is a mix of HWB and EWB concepts. Many experts believe that well-being is a far complex idea than being measured by a unitary basis. The conception of *flourishing* views well-being as a multi-factorial concept as presented by Dr. Seligman in 2013. PERMA – positive emotions, engagement, relationships, meaning and achievement, constitutes not only subjective well-being but also strengthens physical and mental aspects.

Similarly, in 2002, Keyes offered the term *flourishing* to

describe a condition characterized by high levels of both EWB and HWB.

However, all these theorists have only built upon and deeply analyzed the raw theories of Aristotle, Plato and other philosophers; way before social sciences was a thing. "Every craft and every line of inquiry, and likewise every action and decision, seems to seek some good." -- Aristotle

In this statement, the unspecific measure of goodness is an indication of development and psychological growth. It highlights the fact that each action or decision aims for 'some' good meaning there is room for more and as human virtue entails, it will always pursue perfection.

Moreover, the Ethics by Aristotle uses 'well' and 'good' as a description for well-being rather than beneficial or advantageous. Known for his precise use of terms, Aristotle leaves a thought-invoking point for theorists to discuss. Repeatedly, Aristotle emphasizes on 'living well' and doing well' which deduces that if someone is living well, they are living in a good way which is commendable. In contrast, if someone is living as they ought to or what is good to them, it does not always qualify as a complement but highlights a more selfish nature. This shows that

Aristotle's take on well-being was more inclined to EWB measures. However, what's more interesting is the question: Did Aristotle mean that possessing virtuousness is the highest quality of a human or if virtuousness is of highest benefit to humans?

This flows into a very delicate difference between happiness and well-being. The fine line between the two has many overlapping areas often making it hard to distinguish one from the other.

Happiness may not always a measure of your well-being and well-being does not always ensue happiness. A simple example is that a child feels happy when they don't get any homework and get to play video games all day but it is not good for their well-being because it is not allowing them to learn, grow and become healthy. Similarly, drugs give a high level of euphoria but we are all aware that its consumption has severe addictive properties and long-term adverse effects on health.

That is why it is important to constitute elements of happiness separately from well-being. Many people enjoy eating fatty and junk foods but the current rates of obesity and the co morbidities associated are clear evidence how overall well-being is being compromised. However, this does not mean that happiness should not be used as a measure. Why do we say pursue the career that you enjoy? Because the happier you are the healthier.

Different Types of Well-being

The various aspects of well-being allow us to define it within four spheres. This categorization lays the foundation for studying correlation with the vast number of factors affecting well-being. How trauma affects physical health is different from emotional well-being.

Well-being has different types, and there are hundreds and thousands of researchers studying these different disciplines. These include all of the listed below:

- **Physical Well-being**

Physical well-being includes taking care of your bodily requirements like keeping within the BMI standards, eating a balanced organic diet, working out and exercise. A better physical well-being is bound to increase both EWB and HWB.

- **Emotional Well-being**

Amongst all the well-being types, emotional well-being is the most challenging to tackle for most people. The taboo around negative emotions is the greatest barrier. Emotional well-being is the innate ability to accept and address emotional changes be it good or bad. Emotions like sorrow, anger, regret, happiness, excitement, love even lust should be accepted so that you know how to control them.

- **Social Well-being**

Personality disorders are a manifestation of poor social well-being. Social well-being is an important determinant of how one behaves, responds and interacts with other people. Relations, friendships, business contacts are all encompassed in this aspect. This is where childhood trauma, family relations and romantic relations affect our well-being.

- **Mental Well-being**

The most controversial and abstract nature of well-being is mental well-being. Mental well-being mostly comes in consideration when stress, anxiety and depression settle in. in fact, mental well-being is the ability to feel motivated, engagedand focused towards whatever you do.

- **Theories of Well-being**

The various claims and studies on well-being revolve around three core theories of well-being that explain the intrinsic nature of humans that sets the measures and scales for well-being.

- **Hedonism**

Simply put, hedonism is the positive balance of pleasure over pain. Some points of hedonism state that happiness or pleasure is valuable irrespective of their worldly value or virtue. Secondly, unlike popular opinion, hedonism does not refer to indulgent or reckless pleasure-seeking. This flows into the third point that states hedonism as a selfless well-being distinguishingit from egoism.

- **Desire Satisfaction Theories**

In contrast to hedonism, desire satisfaction theory assigns value to things not by a measure of pleasure or happiness but by desire. I want a Tesla or I want to travel the world. This is a desire but to get there you might have to save a lot, work harder, maybe cut down on other activities which is not always enjoyable but the feeling of a satisfied desire boosts well-being. Many theories state that the more desires satisfied, the better the overall well-being of that individual is.

- **Objective List Theories**

The objective list theories focus on things that affect an individual's well-being without being pleasurable or desired. For example, knowledge, health, virtuous behavior. These are all objective. We don't desire knowledge generally nor is the entire process very exhilarating but it is a determinant of our well-being.

Such theories negate the previous two monistic theories that stand upon a single element of well-being. Theorists that support this standpoint believe that life is far more complicated than that. However, this set of theories bring certain concerns to the table. If there are more than one factor affecting well-being there must be a common root from where all these factors branch and if there is why is it not replaced for all the other factors. If there is no characteristic feature in common then why the items on the list are there and why aren't others present too?

Importance of well-being

We keep expounding upon well-being, its factors, its co-variates, the different theories to the point that for centuries theorists have been studying it to formulate the most accurate depiction of well-being. Why is it so important?

Our sense of well-being is essential to our health and generalsatisfaction. Having a robust and well-adapted sense of well- being can assist us in overcoming adversity and achieving our life goals. Enhanced well-being has been associated with increased health advantages, such as lower rates of heart disease, strokes, sleeping disorders, and increased productivity and creativity in both work and personal life. In short, a sense of well-being enables us to be our best selves.

Better mood

Do you work better when you're sad or when you're feeling constipated? No, right? An overall better well-being uplifts your mood. You are more proactive and positive about life referring back to the theory in which positive illusions tend to create better satisfactory outcomes and greater levels of happiness.

Higher functionality

When you're fit and healthy overall, your capabilities are extended; you are working at your best.

Creativity and innovation

Artists and musicians are those that fuel their passions with well-being. Creativity and passion are free and wild and if you're already chained down by your deteriorating well-being, it's impossible to fly with your dreams.

Mindfulness

To be aware of your surroundings, to be vigilant and accountable for your actions is not always an easy task. A healthy well-being clears the cloud allowing you to see what youare and how you present yourself.

Feeling of fulfillment

The current generations h a v e a prevalent trend of feelingempty and unaccomplished despite doing pretty well in life. This is an indication of lacking well-being and surfaces as intangible feelings of emptiness. To feel proud of yourself, you must alignour desires with your actions as stated by the Desire SatisfactionTheories.

Emotional management

Amongst the most prominent advantages of good well-being is emotional management. People that lash out violently in anger are victims of poor well-being. People that feel hollow and unexpressive when hurt or sad have never learned to cater their well-being in all aspects.

Motivation

A flourishing well-being is a motivating element. As stated by Aristotle, some good will always continue until it reaches 'the good' which is perfection. This means that when you feel good or live well you're automatically motivated to be better.

How Do You Measure Well-being?

If we drill beyond the definition of well-being, it's hard to identify what it means in day-to-day life and the right way to measure it.

We resist relying on more traditional mental health measurements, such as sickness symptoms while supporting persons with mental health concerns. Many people who use mental health care services believe that these treatments are outmoded and don't reflect their personal sense of well-being. Many other elements that are majorly overlooked can affect health or happiness. We must also take into account how a person's internal resources (such as positivity, tolerance, and self-esteem) and external situations (such as income, accommodation, and social networks) can affect their well- being. In this regard, measuring well-being is both challenging and rewarding.

There is no 'one size fits all' scenario with well-being, and it can be measured in different ways. However, there are a few effective and valuable ways to measure well-being: WEMWBS, which is the Warwick-Edinburgh Mental Well-Being Scale. This is a 14-item scale with positively worded items intended to assess both the emotional and functional components of positive mental health. For instance, the scale includes statements such as 'I've been positive about the future, 'I've been thinking clearly,' and 'I've been curious about new things.' Participants are asked to select the response that best characterizes their experience with each item over the last two weeks on a five- point scale. The final score ranges from 14 to 70, with a higher number indicating greater well-being.

This measure shows improvement or decline in well-being

over time both at individual levels and overall compared with national averages. It is essential to balance people's perceptionsof their own well-being with life quality indices such as health, daily fitness, and social contact. This information enables you to have the broadest possible perspective on someone's general health and ability to function daily.

Ryff Survey is a variable length survey that allows researcherto study six-point views of a candidate. Based on the details wanted, the items may increase or decrease on the scale.

NHANES (National Health and Nutrition Examination Survey) is a general well-being schedule and allows to find correlation between different variables.

NHIS (National Health Interview Survey) is a measure for global life satisfaction and looks at well-being as a whole whilealso taking in account the quality of well-being.

SPANE (Scale of Positive and Negative Experiences) is typically a brief 12-item scale that studies functioning in important areas like self-esteem, meaning of life, optimism, purpose etc.

The two most important aspects of well-being discussed in this book are physical and mental well-being. **Physical well- being** refers to maintaining a healthy lifestyle that helps us get the most out of our everyday activities without becoming excessively tired or stressed. **Mental well-being** combines emotional, psychological, and social well-being. It influences how we think, feel, and act. It also helps determine how we cope with stress, relate to other humans, and make decisions. Mental health is fundamental in every phase of life, from childhood to adulthood.

Know Where You Stand

Once you know where you stand on that well-being scale, it'll become easier for you to live your life because you'll know which way to go. There are some symptoms that can help you identify disturbed mental health. These can include:

- Having low to no energy

- Feeling helpless and hopeless

- Having unexplained aches and pains

- Pulling away from people and usual activities

- Having persistent thoughts that cause discomfort

- Feeling on edge, worried, and scared

- Thinking of harming yourself

- Experiencing severe mood swings affecting your everyday routine

Take the First Step

Are you willing to make a change in life but don't know where to start? That's understandable. Even if you think you've got an amazing well-being status, there's always room to improve. You can never be the best version of yourself, but you move towards a better, upgraded version every day.

The first step makes all difference. Start working on your physical and mental well-being and everything else will follow. This book explores every single aspect of both of these well- being disciplines and takes you through a journey of staying positive, physically active, productive, and realizing your full potential.

So, let's begin.

PART 1
PHYSICAL WELL-BEING

CHAPTER 2

AN INTRODUCTION TO PHYSICAL WELL-BEING

Physical well-being is a term that is often misunderstood. Most people believe that physical well-being is only related to physical appearance, or we can say the physical health of the body. However, that is not the right explanation. Physical well-being is something that is about the overall health of a human. It is about maintaining a healthy lifestyle that allows us to make the most out of our daily activities.

It basically helps the body to stay away from physical stress and undue fatigue. So, in order to achieve physical well-being, we must take care of our bodies, and that can be done by recognizing our daily habits and replacing them with healthier ones. It is necessary to have habits and behavior that have a significant positive impact on our overall well-being, health, and quality of life.

Those who have the best physical well-being wake up full of energy every day. They don't feel demotivated at work; in fact, their productivity levels are insane. They feel confident enough to handle whatever challenge comes their way. Not only this but words like discomfort, headache, fatigue, and pain are alien to them. Such people have a clear picture of the life ahead of them and they don't struggle to find the meaning of life.

Phrases like "I am too busy with work that I don't get time to have meals on time" or "I am not young as I used to be" can be tempting to some people, and they might feel proud of them for being so busy in their life that they don't get time to even think about their physical well-being. But in reality, this carelessness is eating them from the inside. It is taking away their ability to perform better. They might not feel it at the moment, but after a few years, the signs of poor physical well-being will start showing.

We can understand this concept better through the example of two friends. Both of them belong to the same social background. They have been through the same school and have achieved somewhat the same grades. Also, their financial conditions are kind of similar to each other. Now when they have graduated from university, they get a job at different companies, on almost the same pay. Despite having so many commonalities, they have one thing completely different from one another, and that is their lifestyle.

Friend A wakes up every day at 6:00 am and mediates. He then goes out for a jog for about 30 minutes and prepares himselfa healthy breakfast that includes eggs, beans, and Jam, after coming home. Following this, he gets ready for work and reaches the office on time. He takes multiple breaks during work to maintain his sanity and to remain productive. After work, he goes out with his friends and then comes home and sleeps around 10 o clock. The best thing about him is that he takes care of what he eats, how much he sleeps, and on top of all, how much rest he gives to his brain.

However, on the other hand, friend B has completely different habits and behavior patterns. He wakes up just half an hour before work and then rushes to his office without even having breakfast. After reaching work, he wastes his time scrolling through social media or gossiping about his colleagues. Then he brings work with him home as he wastes nearly all his time during office hours. And finally, he sleeps post-midnight.

So, after analyzing both these examples, we can say that both these friends will lead to very different destinations later in life. There are more chances for Friend A to achieve financial stability and success. Having a healthy lifestyle will make him lead a physically fit and productive life.

While Friend B, on the other hand, is more likely to suffer because of his irresponsible attitude. Also, an unhealthy lifestyle can deteriorate his health and affect his appearance, strength, happiness, resilience, and ability to achieve his goals.

I think nothing can better exemplify the positive impact of physical well-being as well as celebrities and personalities around us you went down that path. It surely isn't just a coincidence that success only found those with a healthy physical routine.

Amongst many such personalities are people from all fields, be it the film industry or business, be it Hollywood or Bollywood. Jack Dorsey, CEO of Twitter and Square, staunchly follows his workout regime of getting up at 5 in the morning, meditating for 30 min, three reps of seven-minute workouts, and then a cup of coffee. This is how he escapes his 18-hour-a-day work stress.

Mark Zuckerberg, a popular name in the business industry and a rapidly growing business tycoon, reveals his secret to fighting exhaustion and breaking from the monotonous ever- demanding work life with exercise and yoga.

Meanwhile, we have the film industry, which has displayed

how physical well-being is more accountable than any cosmetic procedure for its elegance. Alicia Keys reveals that she regulated her water intake and removed fried foods from her diet to clear up her acne-prone skin. Selena Gomez, singer and actress, despite her chronic illness, maintain her glow with her circuit training workouts and dynamic exercises from Pilates to dancing and hiking. At the same time, we have Bollywood's healthiest and fittest, Akshay Kumar, who has been setting unbeatable fitness goals. Shifting to veganism and home-cooked meals, he has displayed how physical well-being has been his success factor.

Anil Kapoor, aged 63, seems to grow younger each day with his utmost dedication to following a strict workout schedule along with a healthy diet plan. The list goes on and only further cements the importance of physical well-being.

Factors affecting Physical Well-being

Physical well-being is truly an innate ability, and only the actions and decisions you make define it. However, the physical health model encompasses a few key factors that can affect those decisions about your physical health.

- **Socioeconomic status**

The most critical point of argument raised during physical health management is the SES. The financial status of any individual is the first determinant that allows them the margin and facility to address their physical health. It goes unsaid that a middle-class man who has to provide for his family and work two jobs does not have the privilege of working out or sleeping well. Considering he has a family to feed, an organic and restricted diet is an expensive option. Many studies in the US and European countries conclude higher socioeconomic status tends to have a positive relationship with physical health.

- **Educational Status**

Education and awareness play a key factor in defining physical health. An additional four years of education lowers five-year mortality by 1.8 percentage points; it also reduces the risk of heart disease by 2.16 percentage points and the risk of diabetes by 1.3 percentage points. Four more years of schooling lowers the probability of reporting oneself in fair or poor health by 6 percentage points and reduces lost days of work to sickness by 2.3 each year.

- **Genetic disposition**

Your immunity and genetic makeup can also play a major role in your physical health. Your metabolism, immunity, risk of other infections, and resistance to infections can affect how your body reacts to certain foods, exercise, and the environment, which is also key factor for physical health.

- **Psychological status**

Your psychological status has a direct impact on your physical well-being. Those with mental health issues will surely have poor physical health. For example, people with depression always complain about poor health. They often suffer from fatigue, sleeping issues, and above all, unexplainable pains and aches in their bodies due to the signaling pathways in their brains.

United States Centers for Disease Control have given out this study that those with depression or anxiety are more at risk of heart disease and hypertension. So, this study proves that our physical well-being can be affected by the psychological status of our brain.

- **Environmental Factors**

Our environment plays a very important role in our physical well-being. Every single thing affects our health, from the air that we breathe to the condition of the roads on which we drive. Whether it be a natural or a human-caused event, everything can directly or indirectly impact our health. For example, if the city that you live in has poor air quality and you breathe that pollution-filled air, then your lungs will automatically be affected.

Similarly, the effects of climate change increased chemical usage, and airborne diseases are visibly seen in the physical as well as mental health of people around the globe.

Importance of Physical Well-being

We, humans, have multiple roles to play in our everyday lives. We have to strive hard to earn money, keep our friends and family happy, and also take care of our household affairs. However, to do this, we need to be fit both mentally and as well as physically. Below I have explained the importance of having the overall physical well-being in check.

- **Better Quality of Life**

One of the biggest reasons why one should take care of his physical well-being is that it improves the quality of life. Diseases take a backseat when someone is physically fit and eats right. Also, those who are physically fit and are away from the risks of diseases are more likely to live about seven years longer than those who are not very active and have weight on the obese side. This means that staying active and physically fit can prevent or can delay the chronic illnesses that are associated with aging.

- **Higher Self Esteem**

Having better physical well-being contributes to higher self-esteem. Those who are not physically fit or have unhealthy habits don't feel the best about themselves. They have self-image issues, and they look down upon themselves from time to time.

But the moment they start taking care of themselves and incorporating healthy habits into their lifestyle, their self-esteem gets a boost.

However, people with good physical health always look

towards the better side. They don't feel demotivated over minor setbacks as they believe in themselves. Their higher self-esteem helps them to get up again after every failure. Such people are never hard on themselves and always work towards achieving their goals.

- **Better lifestyle**

Another reason why having good physical well-being is important is that it helps in having a better lifestyle. If you are physically fit, your lifestyle will be seen. You will be more energetic and will try to make the most of your time. You will eat healthily, sleep on time and take care of your mental well- being also. All this is related to having better physical well- being.

If your physical well-being is not right and you are struggling with different kinds of health problems, then your lifestyle will also not be the best. You will spend most of your time in bed, thinking about your health issues, and with time you might also lose the energy to get your tasks done on your own. So, in order to live a healthier life and have a better lifestyle, it is important to focus on physical well-being. There are many different types of well-being, and they are not all focused on the mind.

- **Improved Work-life Balance**

It is very natural to feel tired, angry, and stressed after work. Long hours at work consume your energy and leave you so drained that you can't even think about getting yourself involved in something fun after that. But that is not the case with physically fit people. No matter how stressful work is, they still manage to take out some time for themselves. Since they are so energetic, nothing stops them from spending quality time with their family/ friend or indulging in their hobbies.

So, one must work towards achieving better physical well-being as it contributes to countless areas of our lives.

Key Aspects of Physical Well-Being

- **Sleep**

People need a sound sleep of 8 hours every night to remain healthy and alert. However, the youngsters of today underestimate the power of having a regular sleep cycle. They have messed up sleeping schedules which ultimately affect their mental and physical well-being. Though sleeping late at night and waking up during the afternoon will give them ample Sleeping hours, it will leave them unprepared for the next day. It will become extremely difficult for them to get to bed at 10 at night and to attend their classes the next day. In short, it can be said that having different sleeping hours can seriously disrupt the sleep cycle.

Our body craves a regular sleep routine, and if the routine is constantly being disrupted, many negative symptoms can erupt. These symptoms can be memory issues, fatigue, emotional instability, sluggishness, and even an increase in sicknesses.

So, since sleep is one of the key aspects of physical well-being, we must work towards fixing our sleep schedule. The very first thing that you need to do is stick to a consistent sleep routine. With this, I mean that you should be sleeping on the same bed, at the same time, and with the same sequence of activities before your bedtime every day. Also, your wake-up time should be the same. This is the only way through which your sleep cycle can get consistent. Though it will take a few weeks to fully create a consistent sleep routine, once you are able to do it then, there is no going back.

It is important to stay away from stimulating activities hour or two before going to bed. These activities can be playing computer games, social media, television, or doing moderate exercise. Also, one should avoid consuming sugary food/drinks or caffeine before going to bed. Instead, you should consider activities that are calming, for example, listening to slow music, reading a book, or meditation. However, if you must use a screen for these activities, use a filter to reduce blue light.

Also, make sure that there are no screens or electronic devices in your bedroom. Since bedrooms are for resting purposes only, you must let them remain a calm relaxing space. There must be comfortable temperatures in your bedroom, and the lighting should also be a little lower than in other rooms. If your bedroom also acts as your workspace, try to dedicate a separate area for it so that you don't get distracted. A little effort and extra time here can considerably boost psychological cues for sleep.

- **Healthy Eating**

Another key aspect of physical well-being has healthy eating habits. It is widely believed that eating healthily means depriving yourself of all the good foods. Many people think that if they shift to healthy eating habits, they will have to feel hungry all the time and eat only green vegetables for the rest of their lives. However, that is not the case. Eating healthy means consuming all the nutrients that the human body requires. This might include fruits, vegetables, meat, dairy, whole grains, and others.

People with better physical well-being always consume all types of foods but in a specific quantity. They never eat too much or keep themselves hungry for longer intervals as both these things cause negative effects on the metabolism leading to a messed up physical and mental health. So, in order to reach there, one must plan out meals and also drink plenty of water.

- **Physical Activity**

Exercise regularly is one of the most crucial things you can do for your health. Physical activity can strengthen your bones and muscles, help you maintain a healthy weight, increase your ability to carry out daily tasks and improve your cognitive health.

Adults who spend less time sitting and engaging in any level of moderate-to-vigorous exercise reap some health benefits. Physical activity influences your health more than very few other lifestyle decisions.

However, for some people exercising can evoke a variety of unfavorable memories, like drill sergeant personal trainers and terrible gym class in school. But, physical exercise does not always have to be a painful ordeal that is done just for health reasons. Exercise has numerous long-term advantages, yet many people find it difficult to incorporate it into their everyday lives. The secret to maintaining a workout schedule is to select an activity you enjoy and can improve at. Just don't push yourself to do it if you find yoga or spin class dull. There are countless different workout classes and approaches that might keep you interested and motivate you to get better.

- **Hygiene**

In order to maintain physical well-being, we must take care of our hygiene. Hygiene is the action that is taken to prevent diseases and maintain health. This can include daily practices like brushing your teeth, flossing, washing hands, showering, and smelling well. Though these things will not directly keep us healthy, they play a very important role in boosting our mood. It can help us feel good about ourselves, keeping us away from mental disorders like depression.

Additionally, maintaining good hygiene entails obtaining regular checkups, visiting the dentist, and, if you have vision problems, visiting an eye doctor. The majority of people can regularly wash their teeth and take a shower. However, many people put off going to their doctor's appointments due to inconvenience. In the long term, it is much more practical to prevent disease or intervene with early therapy than to completely disregard your health problems.

- **Relaxation**

The conventional perception of relaxation is that it is purely a mental activity with solely mental advantages. Simply said, that is untrue. Stress hormones can produce a range of unpleasant symptoms, including adrenal exhaustion, by causing tension to build up in the muscles, which can result in headaches or back discomfort. In the present times, when everything is so fast forward, people have the pressure of doing well and succeeding in life. However, while having ambition is wonderful, scheduling time to unwind and have fun is crucial for your physical well-being. Everyone benefits from some "me time," whether it's getting a massage, relaxing at home with a nice book, or engaging in their preferred sport.

CHAPTER 3

NUTRITION AND DIET

In the previous chapter, we discussed the physical well-being of humans and how important it is for us to lead healthy and happy life. However, in this chapter, we will discuss nutrition and diet. Most people believe that both these things are the same but in reality, they are not.

Nutrition is basically the assimilation of food materials by living organisms that enables them to maintain themselves, grow, and also reproduce. There are multiple functions served by food to living organisms. For example, it provides our body with the materials that supply energy. However, this energy is then utilized for the absorption and translocation of nutrients. Those nutrients assist the cell materials, for locomotion and movement, for excretion of waste products, and also all the activities that are carried out in the human body.

Additionally, food offers the materials that are needed to create the cell's structural and catalytic components. The specific compounds that living things need as nourishment, how they produce these substances or get them from their environment, and the roles that these substances play within their cells are all different. However, broad trends in the nutritional process and the sorts of nutrients needed to support life may be found in all of the living world's organisms.

However, diet on the other hand is the sum of food that is consumed by humans or other organisms. The word "diet" often entails the consumption of nutrition for weight management or other health purposes. Usually, those people, who are facing some kind of health issue or are going through some therapy for a particular health condition, are asked to have a specific kind of diet. This means that they are asked to consume only those foods that can help them meet their physical needs for that particular disease.

For instance, the diet of a person who has diabetes might be restricted to only those foods and drinks that help him in managing his blood sugar levels. The diet recommended for patients with diabetes includes fibrous and non-starchy vegetables and fruits. Since those foods that have more starch and are rich in carbohydrates cause blood sugar levels to increase, so diabetic patients are asked to avoid them.

Apart from health reasons, diet may also vary according to other factors, such as lifestyle choices and religious beliefs. If we talk about personal choices then people who want to lose weight will cut down on their cabs however if their goal is to get more energy, then they will increase their protein intake. So, it can be said that diet is something that people modify accordingto their own choice and preference.

This brings me to the point that both nutrition and diet are codependent. If the diet is the amount of food consumed by individuals then nutrition, on the other hand, is the process of utilizing that food for metabolism, growth, and repair of tissues. The relationship between diet and nutrition and health is 2-way; health status can be affected by nutrient deficiency and vice versa.

What exactly are Nutrition and Diet?

There are many words that form a favorable meaning on the streets, and they are easily used. However, they contain an extensive meaning thus such words include 'Diet' and 'Nutrition".

Nutrition

Nutrition is the study of food and sustenance, including the nutritional composition of various foods, the number of nutrientsneeded for optimum growth and function, and how this varies across individuals.

The study of what we put into our bodies, with a particular emphasis on the nutrients essential to our survival and well-being, is known as Nutrition. It investigates the biochemical and physiological processes responsible for converting the nutrients found in food into energy or their incorporation into the tissues of the body itself. Nutrients used as fuel by our bodies are carbohydrates, lipids, fiber, minerals, proteins, vitamins, and water. Our bodies also use water as a fuel source. It is necessary to consume the appropriate types and amounts of nutrient-dense meals to keep one's health at its absolute best. An essential partof the study of nutrition science is the investigation of diseases caused by a bad diet and the role that food plays in the beginningstages of the development of chronic conditions.

Lack of proper Nutrition is a major contributor to many of today's most common chronic conditions, including fatigue, digestive issues, food allergies, weight gain, depression, and anxiety. Knowledge of Nutrition and the ability to make educated decisions about one's Diet may help one maintain goodhealth throughout one's life.

What is happening at the cellular level, its effect on our desires, and its role in the development of unhealthy or hazardous food cycles are all aspects of nutrition. By advising patients on what foods to consume and how to implement necessary alterations to their eating routines, nutritionists help their patients achieve various health-related objectives, such as preserving and regaining good health, alleviating the symptoms of illness, and warding off disease.

What to eat and what not to eat (and drink) recommendations are disseminated by the media regularly, and much of it is confused and conflicting. Food fads and quick-fix diets have risen in popularity alongside celebrity chefs and good dining. Since everyone has to eat, everyone has an interest in food, and more and more people are beginning to understand that what you eat has both immediate and long-term effects on your health.

As opposed to traditional medicine, which often just treats the symptoms of an illness, naturopathic Nutrition aims to identify and reinforce the body's natural defenses against illness. Improving a bad diet to treat one ailment frequently results in various additional health advantages, including higher energy, better skin, and better sleep.

Whether you become a nutritionist or not, the information you learn will be vital to your health and well-being, so it's worthyour time to learn as much as you can today.

Diet

A diet is the usual dietary intake of a population or species. One of the most effective definitions of Diet is the foods that make up a person's daily intake. Diet can be better understood ifwe stop using the word as a verb and start using it as a noun. A person's Diet consists of these items regardless of how well or poorly they choose to eat. The ultimate objective is to encourage people to make the best decisions for their health.

A person's Diet is the collection of foods and beverages theyeat daily (or a group). A regulated diet, i.e., one that caters to a person's physiological requirements, may be used to treat or manage a disease or health condition. For example, a diabetic person's Diet may be limited to items that aid in controlling blood sugar. Patients with diabetes should consume a diet rich in non-starchy, fiber fruits and vegetables. Starchy meals are high in carbs, leading to a high blood sugar level if consumed insignificant quantities.

Dieting is the process of regulating an individual's food intake to improve one's health and, more specifically, reducing obesity or what is understood to be an excessive amount of body fat. Many weight reduction strategies include consuming fewer of the three macronutrients that make up the bulk of the average person's diet (outside of water) and provide the body with its principal source of energy: fats, carbs, and proteins. These macronutrients are listed in the following order: Due to an early loss of body water, initial weight loss from energy deficits of 500–1,000 calories per day is very rapid. This is especially true if carbohydrates are restricted during the weight reduction process. However, once the effects of dehydration have passed, any diet plan will result in a rate of fat loss that may be purely related to the calorie deficit that is experienced throughout the diet plan.

Co-relation between Nutrition and Diet

Maintaining a populace's health depends greatly on their Diet and Nutrition. Nutrition is the utilization of food for growth, metabolism, and tissue repair; Diet refers to the total amount of food consumed by an individual. Deficits in essential nutrients can have negative effects on health, and vice versa, illustrating the two-way nature of the interaction between food and Nutrition and health. The goal of dietary guidelines is to encourage a diet that satisfies the nutritional need and to avoid diet-related disorders like dental obesity by providing evidence- based food and beverage recommendations for communities. Nutrients are broken down into two groups, macronutrients like protein, carbs, and fat, and micronutrients like vitamins and minerals, according to the relative amounts each is needed for proper human growth, metabolism, and general health. Although carbs provide the bulk of most people's daily caloric intake, fats are the most efficient macronutrient in energy density. Proteins play crucial roles in the body's development, repair, and overall health as structural and functional components in every cell. Vitamins and minerals, which can be found at modest levels in most diets, are crucial for healthy metabolic function.

How do Diet and Nutrition differ?

Consumers must be aware of the difference between Diet andNutrition. It would be easier for them to adopt a healthy diet if they were aware of what one entails. Consumers who often indulge in subpar diets should be aware of the risks associated with their choices. Getting them to eat better by selecting healthier options is the first step. The remedy to their junk foodand processed food intake is to increase their consumption of genuine, whole foods. Healthy alternatives tend to replace junk food over time. While completely eliminating snacks and sweets is unrealistic, the 80/20 rule can help set a more reasonable target. An individual is well on their road to better health and wellness if they can maintain a balanced diet 80 per cent of the time. Intentional eating is the objective, whether one follows a vegan, low-carb, or Mediterranean Diet.

A person's overall Nutrition can be improved once they make changes to their Diet. They should boost their nutritional intake by opting for organic and locally farmed meals to remedy this. Knowing the nutritional value of your food products and offering that information will go a long way with this demographic. People who want to improve their Diet typically opt for items that include only benign, all-natural substances.

They will choose minimally processed meals rich in antioxidants, vitamins, and minerals.

People's health and longevity can be enhanced via the coordinated efforts of Diet and Nutrition. Choices that improve the Diet and Nutrition of the average client are hallmarks of a good food service company.

Types of Diets

There are many different types of diets that people belonging to different parts of the world follow. However, below I have shared the most famous ones.

- **Mediterranean diet**

Mediterranean diet originated in the southern European states and it primarily focuses on the nutritional habits of people belonging to Greece, Crete, and southern Italy. However, nowadays this diet is prevalent in countries like Spain, Portugal, and southern France.

This diet emphasizes the consumption of beans, plant foods, nuts, seeds, olive oil, whole grains, and fresh fruits as desserts, as the source of dietary fats. Also, consuming a moderate amount of poultry and fish, small amounts of red meat, and low amounts of wine are also allowed in this kind of diet. Basically, the Mediterranean diet consists of up to one-third of fats, with saturated fats not exceeding 8 percent of total calorie intake.

To date, this diet is the most extensively studied diet. There are many reliable pieces of research conducted on this diet that tell about its use for lowering disease risk and improving qualityof life.

- **South beach diet**

The South Beach diet was started by nutritionist Marie Almon and a cardiologist, Dr. Agatston. The prime focus of thisdiet is to control insulin levels and show the benefits of unrefined slow carbohydrates than fast carbohydrates. This dietwas devised by Dr. Agatston devised during the 1990s because he was disappointed with the high carb, low-fat, that was backed by the American Heart Association. He believed that it was noteffective to follow low-fat regimes over a long period.

- **Vegan Diet**

In the vegan diet, a person is not allowed to eat anything that is animal based. This means that the consumption of fish, poultry, meat, dairy, and honey is completely forbidden in this diet. Basically, veganism is more of a philosophy where peopleswitch to plant-based foods for the improvement of their health and other ethnical, environmental, and compassionate reasons.

Vegans have this firm belief that modern farming methods are unfavorable for our environment and also unsustainable in the long run. Also, they think that if plant-based food is made apriority by people then the animals will suffer less, and the environment would benefit. This means that there will be more food in the world and people will enjoy better mental and physical health.

- **Raw food diet**

In the raw food diet, people consume food and drinks that arenot processed. Such foods are mostly organic or we can say plant-based. It is believed by raw foodists people must include about three-quarters of uncooked food in their daily consumption of food. Just like Vegans, raw foodists also do noteat or drink something that is animal based.

There are four main types of raw foodists: raw vegans, raw vegetarians, raw carnivores, and raw omnivores.

- **Vegetarian Diet**

Vegetarians might be lacto-vegetarians, fruitarians, Lacto-Ovo vegetarians, living food diet vegetarians, ovo-vegetarians, pesco-vegetarians, or semi-vegetarians. The majority of vegetarians are lacto-ovo vegetarians, which means that they only consume dairy products, eggs, and honey. Recent studies have demonstrated that vegetarians often have longer life expectancies than meat-eaters, as they have lower body weights,and experience fewer ailments.

- **The Zone Diet**

In the Zone diet, there is a nutritional balance of Carbohydrates 40%, fats 30%, and proteins 30% in each meal. Just like most diets this diet also focuses on controlling insulin levels and reducing body weight. This diet is said to be the bestfor those who are working towards weight reduction or maintaining their current weight. The consumption of fats, unrefined carbohydrates, nuts, and avocados is increased in the Zone diet.

- **Ketogenic diet**

The ketogenic diet is famous for its use as an epileptic treatment. It entails consuming fewer carbohydrates while consuming more fat. It seems counterintuitive, yet it enables thebody to use fat as fuel instead of carbohydrates. To keep the diet's overall focus on fat, a lot of healthy fats—like those found in avocados, coconuts, Brazil nuts, seeds, oily seafood, and oliveoil—are added to the diet.

Through a process known as ketosis, the diet induces the breakdown of fat reserves for fuel and produces compounds known as ketones. For those with type 1 diabetes, the hazards of this diet include ketoacidosis, which can lead to diabetic coma and even death. Although the majority of studies last only two years or less, some encouraging research on the control of diabetes, metabolic health, weight loss, and changes in body composition have been conducted.

- **Atkins diet**

The Atkins nutritional strategy, sometimes known as the Atkins diet, focuses on lowering blood levels of insulin by eating a low-carbohydrate diet. People's insulin levels rise and decrease quickly if they ingest a lot of refined carbohydrates. A decrease in the likelihood that the body would utilize stored fat as a source of energy is caused by rising insulin levels, which cause the body to store energy from the food that is consumed.

As a result, followers of the Atkins diet refrain from consuming them while enjoying unlimited amounts of protein and fat. The Atkins Diet has considerable hazards, despite being well-liked for a while. People who are thinking about the AtkinsDiet should see their physician.

Balanced Diet

While many people run after different kinds of diets to lose weight or lead a healthy life, some prefer having a balanced diet. They consume food belonging to every food group, in a controlled amount so that their body weight is not affected. However, the concept of a balanced diet is still unknown to many people.

A balanced diet is basically the kind of diet in which all the nutritional needs of a person are fulfilled. There are a certain amount of nutrients and calories that the human body needs to stay healthy so having a balanced diet can help a person achieve them going over the recommended daily calorie intake. This means that those who have a balanced diet consume foods from every food group like carbohydrates, proteins, fats, minerals, and fiber.

In this way, people get all the nutrients that are required by the human body to work most efficiently and effectively. However, without a balanced diet, there are higher chances of the human body getting infections and diseases that lead to lowperformance and fatigue. This brings me to the point that those children who don't have a proper diet and don't consume enough healthy foods are more likely to experience growth and developmental issues. Also, such children cultivate unhealthy eating habits that may stick with them even till adulthood. According to the Center for Science in the Public Interest, 4 of the top 10 leading causes of death in the United States are directly linked to diet.

Diet Planning

Diet planning refers to identifying and deciding the usual nutrient intake level. The objective of diet planning, whether for people or for groups, is to have diets that are nutritionally adequate or to guarantee that the likelihood of nutrient excess or insufficiency is as low as is tolerable.

Commercial diets frequently contain nutritionally imbalanced ingredients that result in rapid but temporary weight loss. Depending on the nutrients you are deficient in your diet, these nutritional imbalances may potentially have additional detrimental effects on your health. This can lead to a pattern of yo-yo dieting to maintain weight loss, and this tendency might cause you to gain back what you've lost—and maybe even more.

A balanced diet that has the proper ratios of several macro and micronutrients is crucial. A balanced eating plan promotes long-term, sustained weight loss and ideal health. Six principles are important to be incorporated into a diet plan. These principles are:

- Exploring a varied diet that provides all the nutrients necessary for good health.

- Maintaining adequate levels of nutrients, energy, rest, and movement for optimal health.

- Balancing different food groups, and also eating in the right proportion.

- Consuming an adequate number of calories in order to maintain a healthy weight that is in accordance with your metabolism and exercise levels.

- Focusing on creating a nutrient-dense diet without being high in calories.

- Learning how to be moderate with foods that have higher quantities of sugar or fat.

Importance of a Balanced Diet

The basic aims of a healthy diet are to improve one's state of mind, energy level, physical health, and overall well-being. In order to keep in good health, it is important to eat right, exercise frequently, and stay at a healthy weight. A healthy diet is crucial to your well-being. You can put your health at risk for things like sickness, infection, and fatigue if you don't eat well for your body. Children's vulnerability to a host of growth and development issues may be mitigated, however, by ensuring they consume a diet rich in essential nutrients. The incidence of diseases including heart disease, diabetes, cancer and stroke can all rise in tandem with dietary inadequacies.

As well as improving physical health, regular exercise also has a positive effect on mental health by mitigating negative emotions, including tension, despair, and pain. Physical activity reduces the risk of several health problems, including metabolic syndrome, stroke, high blood pressure, arthritis, and anxiety.

However, people often contradict between having a good diet and having a good meal that gives them a balance. The term 'Diet Planning' narrates the proper mixture of how Diet is to be sustained.

What is Diet Planning?

Diets provide other benefits besides weight loss. Changing your Diet is not only one of the most effective methods of weight loss, but it may also serve as a springboard to other positive behavioral changes, an increased emphasis on your health, and an increase in your level of physical activity.

However, it may be overwhelming to choose a diet plan among the plethora that are out there. For various reasons, many people will do better on various diets in terms of suitability, longevity, and efficacy. The goal of certain diets is to minimize food consumption by reducing hunger, whereas the goal of others is to reduce calorie and carbohydrate intake or fat intake. Some people advocate for changes in eating habits and way of life rather than a strict diet.

Principles of Diet Planning

- These are the six most important principles for diet planning.

- Sustaining a healthy balance between energy use,

nutritional intake, physical activity, and rest is essential.

- Eating a variety of meals in appropriate portions.

- Maintaining a healthy weight by eating enough calories to support one's metabolism and physical activity level.

- Putting forth the effort to develop a diet that is nutrient-rich without being overwhelmingly caloric.

- Develop a sense of moderation while consuming meals that are higher in fat or sugar.

- Trying new foods to find combinations that work to get the nutrients you need to be healthy.

Diet Vs Meal

A diet is a set of rules that control what foods you may and cannot consume, whereas a meal is just a certain amount of food that has been measured out in advance. A meal consists of many courses that are consumed in one sitting (dinner is a meal, lunch is a meal, fish and chips are a meal etc.) The term "diet" refers to the food that is consumed regularly by an individual.

A diet is an ordered plan for what you should consume

regularly, whereas a meal is a fixed amount of food delivered in one sitting. Meals are distinguished from diets by the term "meal."

Types of Nutrients

Generally, there are more than 40 kinds of Nutrients in the foods we consume, however, these nutrients are classified into 7 main food groups that are explained below:

- **Carbohydrates**

Those foods that are rich in carbohydrates are an essential part of a healthy diet. Carbohydrates provide the human body with glucose, which is then converted into energy that helps our body to perform bodily functions and other everyday tasks. However, it is important to understand that carbohydrates must be consumed in a healthy amount as an excess of them can cause serious health issues.

If unhealthier forms of carbohydrates like white bread, sodas, pastries, and highly processed food are consumed then they can contribute to heart issues, diabetes, and also weight gain. Therefore, only the healthier form of carbohydrates like vegetables, whole grains, beans, and fruits should be consumed.

- **Fats**

Fat is the primary energy storage type in the body and is used as a fuel source by the body. A moderate amount of fat is required in the diet for optimal health since it performs numerous other vital activities in the human body. Food contains a variety of fats, such as monounsaturated, polyunsaturated, and saturated fats. It might be unhealthy to consume too much fat or the incorrect kind of fat.

Fats can be found in foods such as seafood, meat, nuts, dairy products, oils, and seeds. Fat is something that helps the human body to prevent heat loss in extremely cold weather. Also, it protects the organs of our body against shocks. Fats make up a part of the cells in our body and are responsible for transporting fat-soluble vitamins such as vitamins A, D, E, and K.

- **Fiber**

Fiber is a type of carbohydrate that is not digested by the human body. Though many carbohydrates that we consume are broken down into multiple sugar molecules, which can also be called glucose fiber on the other hand never breaks down into sugar molecules. It passes through the body undigested and helps in the prevention of constipation. The main sources of fiber are cereals, fruits, vegetables, and oats.

- **Minerals**

Minerals are a class of important minerals that control a variety of bodily processes, including fluid equilibrium, muscle contraction, and nerve impulse transmission. Some elements, like calcium, support bone health and strength as well as body structure.

Minerals can be found in eggs, avocados, shellfish, beans, cruciferous vegetables, organ meats, cocoa, yogurt, cheese, starchy vegetables, nuts, and seeds.

- **Protein**

One of the three macronutrients—nutrients the body needs in greater amounts—is protein. Fat and carbs are the other macronutrients. Long strands of amino acids make up proteins. Since it is found in every bodily cell, consuming enough protein is crucial for maintaining the health of the muscles, bones, and tissues. The main function of protein is to build, repair and maintain healthy body tissues.

Protein plays a role in many bodily processes, including fluid balance, vision, immune system response, blood clotting, enzymes, and hormones. So, it can be said that protein is the kind of nutrient that is important for the growth and development of humans. Meat, eggs, seafood, dry beans, dairy products, grains, seeds, and nuts are good sources of protein.

- **Vitamins**

Vitamin is said to be a kind of nutrient that is required by a human body in small amounts in order to function and remain healthy. Foods made up of animals and plants and also dietary supplements are great sources of vitamins. There are different kinds of vitamins like vitamins A, C, D, E, and K, choline, and the B vitamins (thiamin, riboflavin, niacin, pantothenic acid, biotin, vitamin B6, vitamin B12, and folate/folic acid).

- **Water**

Since water is a necessary nutrient for all life stages, maintaining proper hydration is important for overall health. Asan adult's body weight is made up of around 60% water, whenever we are thirsty, which is the primary warning indication that our body is dehydrating, we consume liquids. Water can be found in foods like cucumber, apples, peaches, watermelon, tomatoes, lettuce, and celery.

Towards the end of this chapter, I would say that having a healthy diet throughout the lifetime supports the normal growth and development of a human. It helps maintain normal body weight and also reduces the risk of serious or chronic health diseases. Therefore, one must pay proper attention to his or her diet and should keep a check on the kinds of food they consume, as this is the only way to lead a healthy and happy life.

Conclusion

Humans have been exercising and researching optimal Diet and lifestyle choices for decades. A healthy lifestyle may be achieved in various ways today, and a diet and nutritional plan will work for everyone, regardless of their unique body composition. However, a balanced diet and proper Nutrition are equally essential for human survival. There are essentials in every Diet and every type of Nutrition. The provision of correct Nutrition with a balanced and nutritious diet may help us feel better. Therefore, it's important to regularly assess ourselves and go over our demands.

CHAPTER 4

CLEAN EATING

Healthy eating involves ingesting various meals that provide the nutrients needed to maintain perfect health, feel great, and be energetic. Protein, carbs, fat, water, vitamins, and minerals are all examples of these nutrients.

A balanced diet is essential for optimal health. It guards you against a broad range of chronic non-communicable diseases, notably heart disease, diabetes, and cancer. Consuming various meals and minimizing sodium, carbohydrates, saturated fats, and commercially produced trans fats are major elements of a balanced diet.

Individual characteristics (e.g., age, gender, lifestyle, and physical activity), cultural context, locally accessible foods, and food patterns all affect the composition of a diversified, balanced, and wholesome diet. A healthy diet is still centered on the same core rules from before.

Everyone should give importance to their diet. When paired with physical activity and moderate body weight, proper nutrition effectively keeps your body healthy and strong. Eat well if you've had any illness in the past or are presently undergoing any kind of medical treatment. The foods you eat can influence immunity, mood, and energy levels.

Benefits of Clean Eating

If you plan to eat healthily, you must have heard of clean eating. But what is clean eating, and what exactly are the benefits of clean eating?

Mainly, it implies consuming whole foods in their natural state rather than highly processed foods with additional sweeteners, chemicals, and additives. Although the specifics vary according to your level of rigidity, the principles of clean eating are straightforward and include foods such as:

Now that you know what kind of food items come with clean eating let's talk about some of the clean eating benefits that you must know before you begin your healthy journey. Clean diet meals are rich in water and include an appropriate balance of minerals and vitamins. Consuming these meals can allow the body to function more efficiently and maintain homeostasis (or optimal balance).

It Helps Improve Your Mood: Clean food is packed with

mood-boosting antioxidants and other good nutrients for your mental health.

Helps with Weight Loss: Because clean foods generally have lower calories than junk food, keeping a caloric deficit is simpler than it is with junk food.

Enhanced Immune System: It provides high antioxidant elements and is mineral-rich, supporting a healthy immune system.

Prevents Aging: Protects against oxidative stress, which is a major cause of premature aging.

Disease Prevention: It helps prevent long-term chronic diseases, including cancer and cardiovascular problems.

Anti-Inflammatory Elements: If you switch to clean foods, they can reduce chronic inflammation associated with many chronic illnesses.

Gives You More Energy: A balanced diet nourishes your body properly and enables you to feel energized and productive.

Better Mental Health: A nutritious diet also benefits your mental health. Certain nutrients in your diet, such as vitamin B-6, contribute to dopamine production, a neurotransmitter associated with pleasure.

Glowing Skin: When you eat well, you obtain more vitamins, minerals, and hydration, reflecting in your skin! Also, it nourishes the skin and nails.

The primary reason to embrace clean eating is the health benefits of consuming foods high in nutrients that have not been extensively processed. Most Americans follow a diet high in packaged foods manufactured with synthetic components and loaded with fat, sugar, sodium, chemicals, preservatives, food flavors, and other additives your body cannot metabolize. These added substances may negatively affect your general health and well-being. Clean eating nurtures your body with nutritional and balanced foods. Clean meals provide your body with an abundance of vitamins and minerals, high-quality protein, and healthy fats, which help your heart and brain, aid in weight control, strengthen your immune system, and boost your energy levels, among other benefits.

Natural foods are far more delicious. While it may seem difficult to consider eating a clean diet, the rewards may far surpass any reservations you may have.

Risk Factors

Did you know that almost half of all adults in the United States, or 46%, consume an unhealthy diet lacking in fish, whole grains, fruits, vegetables, nuts, and beans and excessive in salt, sugar-sweetened beverages, and processed meats? Well, it's true, according to a study report. Additional data indicates that children in the United States are doing even worse: more than half, or 56%, have an inadequate diet.

Under- or overeating, not eating enough of the nutritious meals we need daily, or consuming too many foods and beverages that are low in fiber or heavy in fat, salt, or sugar areall examples of poor eating habits.

Insufficient nutrition can have a short-term impact on our ability to work and a longer-term impact on our chance of getting various illnesses and health issues. These can include:

- Eating Disorders
- Cancers
- Tooth Decay
- High Blood Pressure
- Heart Disease
- Strokes
- Being Obese

- Depression
- High Cholesterol

Nutrition refers to how much and what kind of food one intakes. Nutrients are acquired, processed, and consumed by organisms to sustain all of life's processes, which is what is meant by nutrition. After the body digests the food, it releases the nutrients it requires, such as protein, fat, and carbohydrate. The body cannot function correctly if it lacks these components.

Every human being on the planet has had a basic need for nutrition since the dawn of time. For most people, nutrition is defined as the process of providing the body with the energy it needs to carry out daily activities. Disease, weakness, and disability are all directly linked to a deficiency in food nutrients intake. In addition, the effects of a poor diet might be severe.

Importance of Macros

Many people use calorie counting to keep track of their daily caloric intake to stay on the right path with their fitness goals. Calorie counting is a popular approach. However, another more critical factor is macros, short for macronutrients. On the other hand, micronutrients are vitamins and minerals that the body requires less, such as vitamin C and zinc. Macros help monitor your fitness objectives or just stay healthy in general. To fully have a balanced diet, you must ingest a variety of nutrients that provide fuel to your body and aid in digestion. This can help you achieve your health objectives more quickly than focusing solely on calories. There are three main types of macros:

- Carbohydrates (Carbs)
- Fats
- Proteins

Your body needs these nutrients in large quantities. Regardless of diet plans, you require all three: Eliminating macronutrients increases your chances of developing nutrient deficiencies and sickness.

Carbs: Carbohydrates provide instant energy. When you ingest carbohydrates, your body transforms them into glucose (sugar). It either uses them immediately or stores them as glycogen for later use, which frequently happens during exercise and between meals. Complex carbohydrates, such as starchy vegetables and whole grains, also benefit digestive health due to their high dietary fiber content. Sugar is a simple carb, majorly found in vegetables and dairy.

When most people hear the word *carbs*, they think of bread, cereal, and potatoes. However, the list of carbohydrates-containing foods is relatively long. Complex carbs can be found in food items, such as vegetables, fruits, whole grains, and lentils.

Fats: Your body relies on dietary fat to perform a multitude of roles. You require fat to absorb fat-soluble vitamins (A, D, E, and K), to warm you up in cold conditions, and allow you to spend long amounts of time without meals. Consumption of fat in the diet helps keep your organs healthy, promotes cell growth, and increases the generation of hormones. Since fats have nine calories per gram compared to 4 calories per gram of carbohydrate or protein, they are unfairly judged. On the other hand, healthy fat should be a part of everyone's diet. These include seeds, vegetable oils, fat-containing dairy, nuts, and butter.

Proteins: Protein assists in the development, healing, muscular growth, and disease resistance, to name merely a few of its many benefits. Amino acids are the building blocks of many of your body's components, including proteins. In order to get the 20 amino acids, you need, nine of them are essential, which means your body cannot manufacture them on its own. Among many foods high in protein are poultry, beef, fish, soy, and a selection of dairy products, including yogurt and cheese. Cereals, veggies, and beans are also healthy protein sources if you follow a plant-based diet.

Recommended Macro Consumption

How many macros should you eat? There's no proper answer to this question. Since every human being is different, every person's preferable macronutrient intake is different. Each macronutrient is connected with a specific number of calories per gram:

- Carbohydrates have a calorie count of four per gram.

- Proteins have a calorie content of four per gram.

- Fats contain nine calories per gram.

According to the official dietary guidelines, the suggested daily macronutrient ratio that you should consider in your planning is as follows:

- 20 to 35 percent fats

- 45 to 60 percent carbs

- Remaining protein

Your macronutrient ratio determines your health and fitness objectives and your body's reaction to specific meals. The governmental recommendation is based on the fact that carbohydrates are the body's primary energy source and are the simplest macronutrient for the body to transform from food to energy. The metabolic pathways for fat and protein are considerably more complex and time-consuming, which is inconvenient when you want rapid energy.

How to Calculate Your Macros?

There are several ways in which you can calculate your dailycalorie needs. For example, you can always opt for an online calculator. It's the easiest way to estimate your daily caloric needs. The most popular calculator is IIFYM BMR Calculator. IIFYM's full form is "If It Fits Your Macros," – a popular term used as a hashtag in the macro-tracking fitness communityrelated to flexible dieting plans. All you need to do is use your body and lifestyle information, enter it into the app, and calculate your calorie needs. It considers your daily routines, workout, and other important factors.

Another popular way is to use the Mifflin-St. Jeor Equation.

Here is the equation that you can use:

[We would add the equation image here.]

Once you enter your details into this equation, you multiply the result by an activity factor. For which, you've to use these multipliers that represent your daily activity level:

[picture will be added]

The final figure represents the individual's total daily energy expenditure (TDEE). This is the number of calories they burn on a daily basis. Individuals wishing to lose or gain weight can significantly raise or reduce their caloric intake but should do it gradually.

Your macros are worthless if you don't use them. "Tracking macros" includes the practice of recording all of your meals and tearing down your macro ratio to ensure you're eating in compliance with your goals. This may seem frightening, but the internet comes to the rescue once again with a host of digital macro-tracking apps. Some of these helpful apps include MyFitnessPal, MyMacros Plus, and Cronometer. You can search for them on Google; the packages and all information are readily available there.

While macro tracking might be time-consuming, it may also assist you in achieving your weight or energy goals.

Finding the ideal macronutrient distribution for you may take some time. Consumption tracking can potentially become compulsive and is not suitable for everyone. Consult your healthcare provider before beginning to track macronutrients.

Types of Diets

The reasons for eating a variety of foods are numerous. Eating for health is only one of several considerations that go into our daily meal choices. For ethical and environmental considerations, some people's eating habits are dictated by their medical issues or allergies to specific foods. Their religious or cultural background might influence their preference for one dish over another. As the last point, we all have our own tastes regarding eating. When something works for you, you think everyone should do the same. This is partly due to the media's promotion of the school of thought that there is an ideal way to eat.

There are different types of diets popular today. These include:

Ketogenic Diet (Keto)

If you use Instagram and follow some fitness influencers, Keto is a word you must have heard! The ketogenic diet is an extremely low carbohydrate, high-fat diet that is quite similar to the Atkins and low carbohydrate diets. It entails dramatically lowering carbohydrate consumption and substituting fat for carbohydrates. This carbohydrate restriction induces a metabolic condition called ketosis in your body.

This results in your body becoming extremely effective at burning fat for energy. Additionally, it converts fat to ketones in the liver, which may be used to power the brain.

Ketogenic diets have been shown to significantly lower blood sugar and insulin levels. Along with the higher ketones, this offers a number of health advantages.

Plant-Based Diet

For example, vegetables and legumes should make up most of your diet if you choose a plant-based one. Many people misguidedly believe that a plant-based diet equates to being vegan. Plant-based, however, encompasses a wide spectrum of dietary habits. Plant-based diets may be divided into three categories based on the number of animal products they use in their diets. Some common variations of plant-based eating include flexitarian (semi-vegetarian), pescatarian, vegetarian and vegan.

A widespread misconception is that switching to a plant-based diet can make you healthy right away. Although certain highly processed vegetarian or vegan cuisine is regarded as heart-healthy, these meals are not considered part of a balanced eating plan. Make fresh produce, healthy grains, and minimally processed meals the foundation of your diet.

Mediterranean diet

The definition of the Mediterranean diet varies from country to country and region to region. An old-fashioned way of eating, the Mediterranean diet dates back to the 1950s and 1960s. This area's contemporary cuisine is higher in red meat and processed meals. There are a lot of vegetables, fruits, grains, and legumes in it, as well as fish and healthy fats like olive oil. A heart- healthy diet includes all of these items.

People with a high predisposition to heart disease benefit from lowering their blood pressure, lowering their cholesterol, and improving their blood sugar levels. Meat and dairy products are typically restricted in this diet. Because fewer people eat meat, the saturated fat content is lower. Those who follow this diet are less likely to develop heart disease.

Paleo Diet

Paleolithic humans survived on a range of diets based on what was accessible to them at the time and where they lived around the planet. There is no single "correct" way to eat for everyone. Some opted for a low-carbohydrate, high-protein diet, while others opted for a high-carbohydrate, high-plant diet. In the end, this is only a general suggestion, not a set rule. All of this may be tailored to suit your specific preferences anddemands.

According to the Paleo Diet rule, you should eat meat, eggs, nuts, seeds, spices, herbs, healthy fats, vegetables, fruits, fish, and oils. On the other hand, avoiding food includes artificial sweeteners, soft drinks, grains, processed foods, dairy products,vegetable oils, and trans fats.

How Body Reacts to Clean Eating

The changes our body goes through after it shifts to a clean diet are not what you would expect. People believe that the day they start eating clean, their life is going to seem brighter and healthier. But like any transition, it can be hard and challenging.

Change in the gut microbiome

The first thing that changes in our body is our gut microbiome, and everything that follows is a consequence of this. Our body is greatly dependent on micro-organisms to the point that we are 90% micro-organisms. The gut is where most microbiome is present and is balanced by the food we take in. so based on your diet, you may have your own balance of microflora, and it's not necessary that this balance may always be good. However, when we change our diet, the micro- organism balance changes, and it may take our body time to adjust to it.

Diarrhea or constipation

When the gut balance changes, constipation, and diarrhea is common because the metabolism process shifts and takes time to adjust.

Blood sugar fluctuation

This symptom is usually caused by people who make a

drastic change in diet. Pre-diabetic patients or people with previously risky eating habits may face considerable changes inblood sugar levels. This may cause them some of the symptomsassociated with diabetes, like breaking into a cold sweat, dizziness, etc.

Fatigue

Usually, a clean diet means cutting down on carbs and sugar, especially unhealthy ones. This is why going on a clean diet means that your body will not receive its regular dose of sugars and might initially metabolize fats or proteins. You may get fatigued more easily than usual.

Disturbed Sleep Pattern

The first lifestyle disruption when the stomach is unhappy is your sleep pattern. Your body is stressed and uncomfortable, so you may experience sleepless nights or untimely naps. Often doctors ask about sleep because it can tell a lot about your healthand mental state.

Withdrawals and Cravings

Junk food is considered addictive, and a person can actually face withdrawal symptoms from it. So, when you go from a highcarb diet or pleasure foods to a clean diet, your brain does not produce the happy hormones that are often released in an intoxicated or addicted state. So, you might crave unhealthy snacks once in a while.

Headaches

Headaches follow when you're not getting enough sleep, or you're fatigued, so it can get very frustrating to follow a diet planwith everything else.

However, these are the first few weeks of changing to a cleandiet. This is the time when your body is responding and adjusting to a new lifestyle change. Once you get through these initial symptoms, the body exhibits the detoxifying effects that clean diet promises.

Mental Clarity

Mental clarity is the first thing you experience when the bodyfalls on the track. High carb diets often make you lazy and slow and clouds your mind. But with a clean lighter diet, your mind is not burdened with all the sugars.

Weight Loss

After the first couple of weeks, you might see yourself losingweight, so if you're aiming to lose some, this is the time you tweak your diet and stick to a regime.

Energetic

You will feel more energetic after you let go of the unhealthy lifestyle. With the calories balanced and your body en route, its detoxifying journey allows you to be more productive andactive.

Blood Sugar Improvements

You will notice that your blood sugar levels start falling in the normal range, and if you're diabetic or pre-diabetic, you willnotice an improvement in after-meal sugar levels. This might mean that your body is healing and working on the insulin resistance that had developed.

Positive Mindset

A positive mindset is the greatest benefit and changes you will experience after the irritation and uneasiness of a clean diet. Your body is feeling better after shedding some extra pounds and is now more energetic. The mental clarity does you good tosee life from a positive perspective.

Hormonal Balance

Weight gain and extreme sugar levels are usually the first cause of hormonal imbalance. A clean diet provides your body with all the essential vitamins and minerals like magnesium, calcium, and potassium required for our body's hormonal and enzymatic procedures.

Health Improvement

The long-term changes followed by a clean diet are health improvement symptoms like blood pressure and blood markers. Glucose, VLDL particles, triglycerides, and c-reactive proteins will likely be improved from the starting point.

Making Lifestyle Changes to Complement the Diet

However, it is important to note that the desired effects of a clean diet only become evident when accompanied by other lifestyle changes. It is a common misconception that people want to see health changes with only the diet while continuingwith their risky behavior.

- **Exercise and yoga**

One of the most important lifestyle changes that a healthy diet demands is exercise. The body's requirement for exercise exceeds just physical benefits, but the increased activity uplifts mood and mental capacity. Walking, cycling, jogging, swimming, and even any kind of sports should be included in your daily routine. Similarly, yoga is a generations-old tradition that has been proven to enhance mindfulness and body processes.

- **Drink plenty of water**

This one you might have heard many times. Water is the universal solvent and mediates all body processes. It is essential for our body to consume enough water as it:

- Maintains body osmotic pressure
- Helps in enzymatic and synthesizing processes
- Keeps skin hydrated and firm
- Allows to regulate body temperature
- Helps excrete metabolic waste products
- Monitor sleep routine

As mentioned above, the first few weeks of dieting can subject you to disturbed sleep patterns. Besides that, it is also important for you to maintain a sleep routine. People who work long hours without any rest, spend entire nights partying, or just not sleeping are compromising their health. Having and maintaining a body clock allows your body to be in sync with your routine.

- **Cut down on alcohol and caffeine**

The clean diet obviously calls for a cut down on caffeine

and alcohol. Once in a while is okay, but people who strive on caffeine doses and regular drinking can really interfere with the body's normal detox.

Misconceptions of Clean Eating Diet

Myth#1: Healthy eating and clean eating are the same things

Truth: in principle, healthy and clean eating are not the same. The key difference between both is the limit of consumed packaged or processed foods. According to Harvard University, a healthy eating diet plan generally has the following:

- Daily ample intake of fresh fruits and vegetables, meaning the canned ones won't do.

- Avoid fried foods like fries, nuggets, fried fish, etc.

- Consuming healthy fats and oils with a minimum content of saturated and trans fats.

- Brown pasta and rice in replacement of white rice, sugar, and wheat.

- Choosing natural protein sources like fish, poultry,

nuts, and beans but not bacon and sausage.

- Replacing sugar in your coffee and tea and avoiding artificial and added sugars.

Simply put, healthy eating is not as restrictive as a clean dieting plan which does not make either of the diets better than the other. What matters most is the attitude towards a healthy diet and the extent of restriction required.

Myth#2: Clean eating is always good for you

Truth: People that take clean eating as an obsession may totally miss the purpose of the diet. Eating disorders can be a result of such obsessions where they are fixed on choosing the cleanest foods to the point that they might neglect their body requirements. Scientists call it orthorexia Nervosa, which translates to "fixation on righteous eating."

Although their diet plan is clean, people are so focused on the calorie intake that they may punish or isolate themselves. This is why a clean diet also requires a healthy mindset and attitude towards it. A clean diet should aim to enhance your health standards rather than a restriction or a source of guilt. Such obsessive-compulsive disorders require medical attention to study their cognitive-behavioral trends.

Myth#3: A vegetarian diet is an automatically healthful one.

Lesser unhealthy fats, high vitamins and minerals with all the macros required – seems like a perfect diet. A plant powered diet may seem like the way about it but a healthy diet is not just about what you eat but what you don't eat as well. There are certain nutrients that come from animal sources and are importantcomponents of a healthy diet.

Myth#4: It's healthier to eat egg whites rather than wholeeggs.

Truth: The yolk is where a lot of the nutrition is! I have seenmany people separate out the yolk because they're on a "diet." In actuality, the yolk provides much of the nutrient. As we know, the chick's embryo receives its nutrients from the yolk making it rich in many vital components. the yolk actually contains over40 percent of the protein — and more than 90 percent of the calcium, iron and B vitamins — in a whole egg. It also contains all of the egg's healthy fat-soluble vitamins (A, D, E and K). Plus, that extra fat will help to keep you full and satisfied for longer than you would be with just the whites!

Myth#5: Processed foods are bad.

Truth: processed read-to-serve brown rice are quite different from processed ramen noodles.

We need to realize that we will have to include some processing and packaging into our diet. Not all of us have the luxury of obtaining our whole grain wheat, kneading it and making our own pasta. In fact, it is not processing that we should swear off but learn what extent of processing we should include. This means you need to choose your packaged foods smartly like canned beans, tuna and fish are okay. You can use quick-cooking grains or pre-washed and cleaned vegetables and fruits. It's about reading the labels and knowing that maximum nutrients have been retained.

Myth#6: Calories are bad.

Truth: You need calories to live. The word calories often give out the bad vibes but that's only when they're making home in your arteries and veins. Calories are important for you but when you start focusing on the quality of calories, the quantity will be the last of your worries.

The Snacking Dilemma

You may realize that your clean diet may not always satisfy your hunger and you may resort to snacking. Snacking on a diet is often taken as cheating or extra calories but if you plan your snacks, they can help you maintain your diet, feel satisfied and keep you balanced and calm.

The untimely pangs of hunger between meals often make you "hangry" (hungry and angry) and this can interfere with your normal routine. Your "hanger" can creep up to you when on a clean diet and few healthy, planned snacks can keep you satisfied.

Experiment with Clean Eating Snacks: Portions and Timing

Use your creativity to make some healthy mid-meal snacks. This can include using the leftover of your breakfast so that it's not even a complete meal but is enough to keep your "hanger" at bay.

The trick is to eat in small portions and eating only between breakfast and lunch or lunch and dinner. Eating before bedtime can make you groggy and lazy.

Plan Your Clean Snacks

Snacking may not be all that bad if you include healthy options on the list. Chips, fried foods, chocolates are common snacking options. Instead choose healthy alternatives like:

- Veggies and Hummus
- Fruit and Nuts
- Guacamole

- Daily Shake

How do you begin clean eating?

1.   Cook your own food.

If you really want to control what goes into your body, start cooking your own food. That way you can control the sugars, salt and flavors that go in along with the calorie count. You may not be able to pull-off the recipe that you intended to copy but it'll be worth the effort.

2.   Read the nutrition labels

Cooking yourself is not going to be easy because you will have to include processed foods. As a beginner on a clean diet, reading food labels should be familiar. You need to know what you're adding to your diet and how much of it constitutes to thecalorie count of your food. Labels also tell you what additives, artificial flavors, sugar or salts are present and is the best way to begin cutting down on additional processing.

Food labels with "Hydrolyzed" or "modified" are usually items that are highly processed and "-ose" foods are the ones that indicate added sugars. These are a few things you should look out for on a label. Instead, include ingredients that have whole grain or whole wheat labels. Also keep sodium levels at the least. On average, a body requires 250mg of sodium each day which is way exceeded by our normal diet.

3.   Eat whole foods.

The idea of whole foods is to minimize processing in foods like whole grain and whole wheat have minimal added sugars and preservatives and are least modified. This may decrease shelf life but are healthier on your plate.

Whole foods include lean proteins, fresh fruits and vegetables, full-fat dairy products, unsalted nuts/seeds, dried beans/legumes, and whole grains. In addition to escaping the added and unnecessary junk from being processed, the unrefinedfoods also carry more nutrients and fiber which is essential for your body to function.

4. Avoid processed foods.

Packaged foods are the biggest indication of processing. The thing about processing that makes it so unhealthy are the additional components and ingredients that are not always beneficial.

5. Eat well-balanced meals.

Along with unprocessed foods, you should also know how to balance our diet. You can eat only fresh proteins, but that would not be a healthy diet. Include all kinds of macros and nutrients on your plate so that you have a variety of all essential nutrients. It should provide fiber, antioxidants, vitamins, and minerals.

6. Limit added fat, salt, and sugars.

Clean eating aims to make our diet as organic and natural as possible so eating food in its whole state or natural form is the recommended form. This tends to help you avoid consuming added sugars, salt or any unhealthy fats and ingredients, since clean eating has the intention of eating food in its most natural, whole state, it makes sense that you would want to avoid unnecessary additives, like fat, salt, and sugar, when choosing your food. Fresh fruit should be all the sugar you need once you are on a clean eating track. The more you follow the clean eating lifestyle, foods you once loved, like doughnuts, hamburgers, fries, and more will taste overly sweet or salty. This is because your body and taste buds will be so used to the whole foods in your new lifestyle that these additives will taste needed and even overdone.

7.   Eat 5-6 meals per day.

The best way to limit calorie count is to forget actually counting them and distributing it all over the day. That way you are bound to consume lesser calories because you will be eating at shorter intervals so you won't require larger portions. Forget the concept of counting calories. If you take 5-6 meals per day, you have a greater chance of distributing the components easily. For example, you can intake whole grain foods in the morning. You can eat lean proteins, fats and fruits for lunch. You can intake fats, vegetables, etc. between lunch and dinner and so on. This ensures that you don't over-eat or skip meals keeping you satisfied throughout the day and giving you an extra boost every few hours.

- **Don't drink your calories.**

Smoothies, shakes, juices – these all seem pretty convenient but account for more calories than you may expect. Be mindful of what you drink. It is always better to substitute your drinks with water as much as you can. Because juices and other beverages can make you thirstier, the more you'll want to drink. However, water keeps you hydrated and full. Moreover, soda drinks are the worst thing you can add to your diet. It is a full fructose-based syrup and other added sugars that are of absolutely no health benefit and can affect bone density. Although fruit juices are a healthier option, they lack the fiber and minerals that come from eating fruits, vegetables etc.

Foods to Avoid

As already mentioned before, the foods to avoid in a clean diet are mainly the processed and packaged foods. Foods with high number of additives, sodium, trans fat and overall low nutritional value tend need to be excluded from a clean diet. Such foods add up to empty calories and are associated with negative health consequences. Some foods that we should avoid:

Processed Foods and Ingredients

- Artificial   Sweeteners: Aspartame,
  Neotame, Saccharin, Sucralose, Xylitol,
  Erythritol
- Refined Sugars: Brown sugar, Table Sugar, Corn
  Syrup
- Processed Meats: Hot Dogs, Spam
- Packaged Foods and Snacks
- Candy
- Chips
- Soda
- Alcohol

Foods to eat

Proteins

Protein sources that have the highest content of protein as compared to carbs and fats are considered the most quality proteins. Grass-fed animals are known to produce the best quality of lean meat and dairy products. Some researches have shown that grass-fed animals are lower in fat and higher in vitamin A and cage free eggs are higher in vitamin D and lower cholesterol levels. This proves that organic feed produces the highest quality of food.

The best proteins are high in quality protein (containing more protein than fat and carbs), lean, and loaded with nutrition. For meat and dairy this typically means opting for more grass-fed, sustainably caught and free-range options. And for many people this also means considering more organic proteins. Research
also suggests that organic dairy from grass-fed cows has a more beneficial fatty acid complex, that's higher in heart healthyomega-3s

Here are some excellent protein choices to look for:

Grass-Fed Meat

- 100% Grass-fed Beef and Steak
- Bison
- Elk
- Venison
- Goat
- Antelope
- Lamb

Organic and Free-Range Proteins

- Eggs

- Egg whites

- Chicken

- Turkey

- Duck

- Pork
- Quail

- Goose

- Ostrich Sustainably Caught Seafood

Fatty Fish: Salmon, Mackerel, Anchovies, Sea bass, Sardines, Sablefish, Pompano, Eel, Carp, and Herring

Lean Fish: Tuna, Basa, Cod, Mahi Mahi, Wahoo, Tilapia, Pollock, Halibut, Rockfish, Trout, Bass, Catfish, Flounder, Grouper, Haddock, Pike, and Snapper

Shellfish: Sustainably-Caught Shrimp, Oysters, Clams, Mussels, Lobster, Crab, and Scallop

- Squid Plant-Based Proteins

- Quinoa

- Buckwheat

- Nutritional Yeast

- Mycoprotein (corn based)
- Beans and Legumes: Navy Beans, Pinto Beans, Black Beans, Butter Beans, Fava Beans, Chickpeas,Lima Beans, Black Eyed Peas, etc.

- Lentils

- Green Peas

- Pea Protein

- Edamame and Tofu (Contain Soy)Organic and

Grass-Fed Dairy

- Cow's Milk

- Goats Milk

- Yogurt

- Ice cream

- Cheese

- Cottage Cheese

- Cream

- Sheep's Milk

- Butter

Carbs

Here are some of the most nutritious carb foods broken out by category, including gluten-free and gluten-containing grains. It also contains sweeteners that are less-processed and can be consumed in small amounts.

Gluten-Free Whole Grains

- Rice

- Millet

- Oatmeal

- Air-Popped Popcorn

- Quinoa

- Teff

- Buckwheat

- Amaranth

- Sorghum

- Corn

- Gluten-Containing Whole Grains

- Wheat

- Pasta

- Bread
- Crackers
- Barley
- Ancient Grains
- Cereal GrainsStarchy Vegetables
- Sweet Potatoes
- Yams
- Yucca
- Other Potatoes
- Corn
- Peas
- Beans
- Legumes
- Lentils
- Acorn Squash
- Butternut Squash

Fruit

- Cherries
- Bananas

- 100% Fruit Juice

- Papaya

- Grapes

- Oranges

- Tangerines

- Pears

- Mangos

- Pineapple

- Frozen Fruit

- Guava

- Apples

- Lychee

- Black Currants

- Peaches

- Figs

- Goji Berries

- Dates

- Dried Fruit

Sweeteners

- Agave

- Raw sugar

- Honey

- Maple Syrup

- Coconut Sugar

- Date PasteHealthy Fats

Dressings, cooking oil, butter and sauces are common sources of fat in your diet. However, natural fats are also present in many protein sources. The best fats are extracted from plant- based sources, packaged with other healthy nutrients.

To get the right balance of fat in your diet, make sure you are tracking your macro intake and portioning high-fat foods tomeet your fitness goals.

Here are some great fats to add to your diet:

- Avocados

- Olives

- Cacao

- Coconut

- Tahini

- Peanuts and Peanut Butter

- Nuts and Nut Butters: Almonds, Cashews,Pistachios, Pecans, Brazil Nuts, Walnuts, etc.

- Seeds: Chia Seeds, Flax Seeds, Hemp Seeds,Sesame Seeds, Sunflower Seeds, Pumpkin Seeds, etc.

- Oils: Flax Seed Oil, Sesame Oil, Coconut Oil,Olive Oil, Avocado Oil, and Canola Oil

Promoting Healthy Eating

Diet changes over time, shaped by a multitude of social and economic forces that interact intricately to influence individual dietary patterns. These variables include incomes, food bills (which alter the availability and affordability of nutritious foods), personal preferences and opinions, cultural traditions, and geographical and environmental factors (including climate change).

Thus, maintaining a healthy food environment – incorporating food systems that encourage a diversified, balanced, and nutritious diet – necessitates the collaboration of numerous sectors and stakeholders, including the government and the public and commercial sectors. Governments have a critical role in fostering an atmosphere conducive to establishing and maintaining healthy dietary patterns.

Concluding healthy eating, it's pretty clear that healthy foodhas numerous benefits, it helps in many phases of your life, and not only it impacts the physical health, but also mental health, which will be discussed further. The main benefits of healthy eating acknowledged are a healthy heart, weight loss/gain, better mood, increased energy levels, better brain health, decreased illnesses, and strong bones.

CHAPTER 5

PHYSICAL EXERTION

Exertion means an effort. When you prioritize physical exertion in your life, much good follows. To put it simply, physical strength and vitality are beneficial for everyone. Workout can help every age, young and old. Irrespective of your body shape or BMI, you should maintain a healthy lifestyle by exercising regularly. But, physical exertion doesn't always have to involve weight-lifting and hardcore training in the gym.

Importance of Physical Exertion

To put it in another way, everyone must engage in at least basic physical activity or exercise. People of all ages need to engage in some form of exercise regularly. Physical exercise is important for overall health and should be maintained at all phases of life, regardless of one's physical characteristics. Knowing the benefits of physical fitness and how much exercise you should be doing will help you retain excellent health and enhance your quality of life.

Here are a few advantages that can improve your standard

ofliving if you indulge in regular physical activity:

Saving Money on Health-RelatedExpenses

7 out of 10 fatalities in the United States are attributed to chronic illnesses, which account for 86% of healthcare expenses in the United States, according to the Centers for Disease Control and Prevention (CDC). Some diseases, such as heart disease and diabetes, are unavoidable, but you may lower your chance of developing them by lowering your hazardous behaviors and adopting a healthy lifestyle.

Many health problems and consequences may be avoided if you make healthy decisions, such as exercising regularly. It's a good strategy to avoid going to the doctor. People who spend much time sitting are more likely to get heart diseases and strokes. According to one research, adults who watch more thanfour hours of television each day had an 80 percent increased chance of dying from heart disease.

Improve your health by being more active. It can:

- keep a lower pulse rate

- increase your healthy cholesterol levels

- increase the flow of blood (circulation)

- manage your weight to avoid osteoporosis-related bone loss

It all adds to lower medical costs, interventions, and drug consumption in the long run!

Staying Active While Growing Old

You can participate in various activities that need a certain level of physical fitness if you want to stay active and healthy. As an illustration, climbing a mountain may be an exhilarating experience that delivers a sense of success and the breathtaking views that come with it. Still, not everyone is physically capable of doing so. But even a family outing to the zoo or a trip to the playground might be a challenge for individuals who have been inactive for a long time. As you grow older, staying involved is simpler if you're physically active. A healthy diet and regular exercise can help alleviate stress, anxiety, despair, and rage symptoms. Those benefits of well-being that come with physical activity are well-known. It's like taking a happy pill without any unpleasant side effects. As physical exercise becomes more of a habit for most people, they begin to perceive an improvement in their overall well-being.

Improving Your Health

Physical fitness has several health benefits, like strong muscles and bones. It enhances the respiratory, cardiovascular, and general health of the person. In addition to lowering your risk of obesity, diabetes, heart disease, and some malignancies, being physically active can help you maintain a healthy weight.

Simply put, being physically active is vital for good health and well-being. Encourage your family to be more active, and challenge yourself to fulfill daily and weekly physical activity goals. Pick up healthy, active pastimes like hiking and cycling with your family, and make time to go to the gym regularly. Make physical activity and exercise a regular part of your life, and don't let it end after a week of trying.

Without regular physical exercise, your body's strength, stamina, and functionality degrade over time. You don't stop moving because you're becoming old; you get old by not moving.

Health Benefits of Physical Activity

Improves Energy Level

Physical activity improves your energy by strengthening the efficiency of your cardiovascular system. You can be more active and perform multiple tasks in less time when you have more energy.

Strengthens your Muscles

Physical exertion strengthens your muscles and makes your joints, tendons, and ligaments flexible. This enables you to move easily, avoid injury, and reduce the risk of back pains by keeping the proper alignment of joints. Furthermore, it also improves flexibility and balance.

Maintain Healthy Weight

The amount of physical exertion is directly proportional to the calories you burn. This allows you to maintain a healthy weight. Also, your metabolic rate increases with physical activity. When you maintain a healthy weight, it makes you physically stronger and boosts your self-esteem.

Strengthens Heart Muscle

Physical exertion is good for your heart as it reduces your heart's LDL cholesterol and increases HDL, the good cholesterol. This reduces blood pressure and lowers the stress on your heart. In addition, it strengthens your heart muscle. If you have a healthy diet and do regular exercise, it minimizes your risk of developing coronary heart disease.

Lowers the Risk of Type 2 Diabetes

Regular physical exertion lowers your risk of developing type 2 diabetes by controlling blood glucose levels. Obesity, a primary cause of type 2 diabetes, is also controlled due to exercise.

Improves Immune System

Physical exertion strengthens the ability of your body to pump oxygen and nutrients around your body. It enhances your immune system and improves the ability of your body to pump blood so that the cells can fight bacteria and viruses.

In addition, exercise minimizes the chances of developing any kind of degenerative bone disease. Physical exertions like running, walking, or weight training reduce the risk of osteoarthritis and osteoporosis.

Reduces the Risk of Cancers

The risk of getting colon, breast, lung, and endometrial cancers is greatly reduced if you are fit and continuously indulged in physical activity.

According to a study conducted by Cancer Research Centre, 35% of cancer deaths result from obesity and inactivity. Exercise improves your physical well-being and is also beneficial foryour mental health.

Improves the Quality of your Sleep

After getting tired due to physical exertion, people tend to sleep better. Sleeping well also improves your physical and mental well-being and reduces stress, anxiety, and depression.

Uplifts your Mood

Physical activity uplifts your mood and improves your self-esteem. It stimulates the release of endorphin hormones, making you feel better and relaxed and calming your nerves.

Help Treat Mental Illness

You must indulge in physical activity if you are frustrated, stressed out, or depressed. It will help you cope with frustration and depression and make you realize your self-worth. In addition, it will give you a sense of achievement and provide you with essential *me time*.

Helping You Live Longer

The new 60 is 70, but only if you're fit and in good physical condition. Overweight and inactive people have a life expectancy of seven years less than those who are physically active and have healthy weights. On top of that, those extra years are often filled with better health. Preventing or delaying chronic diseases and disorders related to aging can be achieved by regular exercise. As a result, active individuals enjoy higher levels of well-being and self-sufficiency as they get older.

Physical activity can provide several other advantages, including the following:

- It increases your stamina and productivity

- It makes it easier for you to deal with stress and

tension

- It helps to cultivate a positive view of life

- It makes it easier to fall asleep and stay asleep

- It helps you to improve your self-esteem and self-image

Different Types of Physical Exertion

Physical exertion plays an important role in an individual's physical and mental well-being. Different types of physical exercises have diverse health benefits. Here are some of the different types of physical exertions that you can do:

Aerobic Activity

Aerobic activities like dancing, bicycling, and swimming improves your heart rate, increasing the amount of oxygen your heart and muscles receive. Such activity is highly beneficial for your heart and muscles. It also uplifts your mood, enhances your self-esteem, gives you more energy, and lowers your blood pressure, cholesterol, blood sugar, body fat, stress, anxiety, depression, and exhaustion.

Muscle-Strengthening Activity

Muscle-strengthening activity, also known as resistance training, helps maintain and strengthen the muscles, endurance, and power. Lifting weight machines, free weights, and Pilates are examples of muscle-strengthening activities. It is pertinent to mention that even activities like lifting children, carrying heavy goods, and climbing stairs come in muscle-strengtheningactivity.

Flexibility Training Exercises

Stretching your body to increase flexibility improves your overall physical strength to perform other types of exercises. Yoga and Tai Chi are examples of dynamic stretches done with movement while holding a position for a few seconds or longer in static stretches without movement. If you use an external force to hold a pose, it comes in passive stretching, while if you do it without an external force, it is active stretching.

Balance Training

Balance training exercises like standing on one foot and walking heel-to-toe in a straight line improve body control and stability. Such exercises require a lot of focus and dedication.

Safety While Exercising

Physical exertion is important for your mental and physical well-being, but so is your safety when exercising. Exercises can result in minor injuries like strained or pulled muscles, ankle sprain, knee sprain, inflamed tendons, etc. In rare cases, vigorous physical activity can even lead to a heart attack or sudden death.

You must consult your doctor first if you are new to exercise or have an illness. Your doctor will be better able to guide you if an exercise is safe for you or not.

Similarly, sometimes, if you try doing too much physical activity, it can negatively affect your heart, muscles, and joints too soon. It can result in injury. Thus, it is important that you start with light exercises shorter in duration and then slowly progress towards more vigorous and intense exercises.

Tips to Stay Safe and Active

Physical exertion is important, but your safety is equally important. So, we will share tips that you can use to stay safe and active.

- If you are pregnant or have any other medical complications, consult your doctor before starting toexercise.

- If you have been inactive for the longest time, don't indulge in heavy physically exerting exercises immediately. Go for lower impact, light to moderate effort exercises like walking, gardening, and slow swimming. Then you can gradually progress from there.

- It is important to protect yourself while indulging in physically exerting activities. For instance, if you are cycling, wear a helmet. If you are going out for a walk, don't wear uncomfortable shoes. Wear sneakers or flip- flops. If you go to a gym, buy gym clothes and use them.

- Use safe and secure places to work out. Go to a family park for walking or a well-maintained gym for physical exercises.

- Don't get into any kind of physical exertion if the weather is too hot or too cold. If the temperature is hot,

- go out for a walk early morning or late evening when thetemperature is cooler.

- Don't ignore signs like nausea, dizziness, muscle cramping, and heavy heartbeat. Just sit down and relax immediately if you go through any signs.

- Keep yourself hydrated. When physically exerting yourself, your body needs to be constantly hydrated, as you release a lot of water in the shape of sweating. For normal workouts of around an hour, drink 24 ounces of water during and after exercising.

- Your diet should complement your exercise. To maintain a healthy lifestyle, you must take adequate amounts of protein, carbohydrates, vitamins, and minerals.

- Be aware of supplements. Fitness trainers often recommend taking supplements to improve your health. But they can be harmful to your body as well. So be aware before taking.

- Observe and listen to your body. If you have signs of fatigue, pain, or lightheadedness, stop physically exerting yourself and take some rest.

How Being Stationery Can Be Detrimental to Your Health

Health complications might arise from a sedentary lifestyle. You have a higher chance of living a long and healthy life if youspend less time sitting or lying down.

You have a decreased chance of early death if you stand or walk around during the day rather than sitting at a desk. Being overweight, acquiring type 2 diabetes, or having a heart attack are more likely outcomes of a sedentary lifestyle, as are feelings of sadness and worry. Humans are designed to be upright creatures. Having a well-functioning heart and cardiovascular system is better for you. When you're upright, your bowels work better, too. People bedridden in the hospital are more likely to have issues with their bowels. In contrast, your energy levels and endurance increase when you engage in regular physical activity, and your bones remain strong.

More than three million people worldwide die each year because of a lack of physical exercise, accounting for six percent of all fatalities. In terms of non-communicable illnesses, it is thefourth most common cause of mortality in the United States. Also, breast and colon cancers account for between 20 and 25 percent of instances and 27 percent of diabetes, and 30 percent of ischemic heart disease. As a matter of fact, physical inactivityranks right behind cigarette use as the leading cause of cancer inAustralia's population. According to the 2011–12 Australian Health Survey results, sixty percent of Australian people do not meet the recommended 30 minutes of moderate-intensity physical activity daily.

Being Stationary for Long Periods Can Lead to The Following Problems:

Weakening of Legs and Gluteal

Your legs and gluteal muscles weaken if you sit idle for a long time. These muscles are important for walking and balancing you. If they become weak, a small injury can becomeworse.

Weight Gain

Being stationary makes you lazy and impacts your digestion,resulting in weight gain. Continuous movement or walking helpsyour body digest food.

According to the latest research, we need 60 to 75 minutes

of moderate to intense activity to fight the dangers of excessive sitting.

Weakening of Hips and Back

Your hips and back will stop supporting you if you sit for long periods. Sitting will cause your hip flexor muscles to shorten, leading to issues in your hip joints.

In addition, if you sit for long periods, especially with the wrong posture, you will also start having back issues. The wrong posture can result in poor spine health and cause compression in the discs in your spine. This often leads to premature degeneration, which is extremely painful.

Anxiety and Depression

People who sit more develop high levels of anxiety and depression. This is primarily because people sitting more are not doing any physical activity and are missing out on the positive effects of fitness and physical exertion.

Increased Chances of Developing Cancer

New studies have found that people who tend to sit idle have higher chances of developing lung, uterine, and colon cancer. However, the reason for it is unknown.

Heart Disease

Sitting idle is linked to heart disease. According to a study, men who watch 23 hours of television per week have 64 percenthigher chances of dying from cardiovascular disease than men who watch 11 hours of television per week.

According to some experts, people who sit a lot are at 147 percent higher risk of suffering from a heart attack or stroke.

Diabetes

According to studies, lying in bed for five days can cause increased insulin resistance in your body. People who tend to spend more time sitting are at 112 percent higher risk of diabetes.

Varicose Veins

Sitting for a long period causes blood to pool in your legs, leading to spider veins or varicose veins. This isn't really dangerous, but sometimes it can lead to blood clots that can be serious.

Deep Vein Thrombosis

Sitting for a long period can also lead to deep vein thrombosis, a blood clot that forms in the veins of your leg.

This is a serious problem because if part of a blood clot in the leg veins breaks off and travels, it can cut off blood flow to the rest of the body. In a complicated situation, it can even lead to death.

Stiffness in Neck and Shoulder

Sitting idle for long periods of just sitting in a bad posture using the laptop can cause stiffness in the neck and shoulders. This can be quite irritating and frustrating.

How to Save Yourself from Dangers of Sitting?

If you're not getting sufficient activity in your day, it's not too late. You can try to gain great health benefits in the process.

• To save your health from the dangers of sitting, try and be more active throughout the day.

• You can start walking or cycling instead of driving all the time. Start using stairs instead of a lift or escalator. If you go on the bus to your desired location, get off the bus a stop early and walk the rest of the way. Park some distance away from wherever you are going and walk the rest of the way. You can also join a gym to indulge in physical activity but go there regularly.

• If you go out for work, you can develop ways to remain active there. Take stairs to work instead of the lift. Walk around with colleagues, go out for lunch and roam around outside.

• Even if you stay indoors, you can remain active by adopting activities such as dancing, swimming at an indoor pool, doing yoga, Pilates, practicing martial arts, squash, etc.

• Reduce inactivity by watching less television, taking a break from work, walking around while attending phone, doing activities while standing up, cleaning around the house, working in the garden, and standing instead of sitting while using public transport.

• If you have just started exercising, and a 30- minute or an hour workout is challenging, then split it into two or three sessions. Remember, it is your effort that counts. Don't overburden yourself, as doing too much too soon can do more harm than good. But again, don't stop doing it completely either.

• Also, don't set long-term goals—set short-term goals, and when you achieve those short-term goals, reward yourself. Positive acknowledgments will build confidence as you commit to achieving fitness goals.

Early Research Linking Illness and Sitting for A Long Time

In 1950, the first link between illness and sitting emerged when researchers found that double-decker bus drivers were twice as likely to have heart attacks as their bus conductor colleagues. This is because drivers just sat 90 percent of their shifts, while conductors climbed almost 60 stairs each day.

It was then found that excessive sitting slows down the metabolism, negatively impacting our blood sugar and blood pressure and weakening muscles and bones.

Further Research

According to an analysis of thirteen studies, people who tend to sit idle for more than eight hours per day with no physical activity are at risk of dying, similar to the risk of dying from obesity and smoking. On the other hand, some other studies found out that if you sit idle for too long, it can be countered with 60 to 75 minutes of moderate to intense physical activity.

Even though a more in-depth study is required to understandthe effects of sitting for long durations, it is clear that the more you move and do physical activity, the better your physical andmental health.

You can break the routine of sitting idle for long periods by standing and walking a bit every 30 minutes, standing while talking to someone, or watching television. It is important to be in motion throughout the day for better health.

It is important to note here that humans are built to stand upright. This way, your heart and the cardiovascular system operate more efficiently. In addition, your bowel also operates better when you are upright.

Conclusion

It is all about your willpower to make your health your priority. Indulging in physically exerting activities can help you grow physically, mentally, and emotionally. You will feel stronger and prouder about yourself. It also helps people love themselves and prioritize their happiness over other things. As it makes you healthier, it gives you a feeling of self-worth and self- accomplishment and minimizes insecurities.

PART 2

MENTAL WELL-BEING

CHAPTER 6

MENTAL WELL-BEING

How we handle the highs and lows of life is a major factor in determining our mental well-being. This straightforward explanation of mental well-being conceals a richer meaning with important repercussions for our daily lives. It encompasses a person's way of thinking and how they manage their feelings (emotional well-being) and behavior.

Our mental health is an essential component of our entire physical well-being. It is common for people in our society to conceive of health in terms of something biological and physical, such as the state of our bodies, the quality of the food we consume, and the amount of physical activity we get. However, this does not account for a significant aspect of one's health. It refers to our mental health, which considers both the inner workings of our minds and how we define where we are in our lives.

Despite the ups and downs of life, a person is considered to be in a state of mental wellness when they prosper in several facets of their life, such as in their relationships, at work, when playing, and in other activities. The realization that we are not our issues and the conviction that we can solve them are necessary components of this state of mind.

Mental Health

"Mental health" refers to an individual's or community's emotional and psychological stability level. A person's mental health, at its core, is measured by how well they can carry out the activities of everyday life, build positive personal and social relationships, grow to their full potential, succeed in school and their chosen career, and make positive contributions to their society. The state of our health directly affects our capacity to reason, socialize, and shape our immediate surroundings. It's the basis for establishing a life of good health and happiness. The right to get care for mental health issues is a cornerstone of human dignity. Furthermore, it is essential for the growth of the individual, the group, and the whole community.

No mental ailment is required for a person to be considered mentally well. These characteristics define it; it exists on a continuum, with different manifestations in different people, causing different levels of suffering and difficulty and having different potential social and therapeutic effects.

Conditions that impact mental health range from ychosocial impairments and mental disorders to states of mind linked with considerable pain, functional impairment, or the likelihood of self-harm. Although it's not always the case or a given, people with mental health disorders tend to experience poorer states of mental well-being.

The Distinction Between Mental Health and Wellbeing:

Imagine the term *"mental health"* in the same way that you would the term *"physical health"* — everyone resides somewhere on a continuum. On the one hand, we have everyday health, which includes nutrition, exercise, and sleep; on the other hand, we have physical problems that may be diagnosed. Similarly, there is mental health, which we all experience daily (stress, anxiety, mood swings, etc.), and mental health disorders, which include but are not limited to bipolar disorder, borderline personality disorder, post-traumatic stress disorder, and depression.

When people talk about "well-being," they are most typically referring to our daily experience of mental health, such as working stress, feeling burned out, or going through an emotionally challenging time, rather than the whole range of mental health, which encompasses illnesses. This is because when most people speak "well-being," they refer to our daily mental health. These are things that every one of us has experienced at some point in our lives; thus, we can all connectto them.

We can also do fundamental things to promote our wellness,such as finding time in our schedules for self-care, taking care of our bodies by maintaining healthy eating and exercise routines, and establishing boundaries in our personal and professional lives. Low wellness can occasionally lead to mentalhealth disorders; therefore, it is always worthwhile to speak outto your support network or a professional if you are struggling if you are having difficulties.

Factors Affecting Our Mental Well-Being:
The things that have happened to us in life, as well as our biological make-up, impact how we think, feel, and respond to the many opportunities, difficulties, and experiences we encounter throughout our lives. How other people treat us, our financial condition, the quality of our relationships, the environment in whichwe work, the transitions that occur in our lives, and even our physicalhealth may all impact our mental health. Certainly, we will all be putin stressful situations at some point in time; nevertheless, the degreeto which we can adapt

to and triumph over these challenges determines the state of our mental health.

Negative Factors:

Negative Social connections: The connections we have with theother individuals in our lives are an essential component of living. We may experience feelings associated with grieving if we are involved in a disagreement or lose one of our connections. Even when surrounded by other people, one might still feel lonely andisolated due to the negative effects of loneliness on one's mental health. It is becoming more difficult to overcome our emotions of loneliness due to the ongoing epidemic and the attendant social constraints that have resulted from it. To continue learning about the effects of loneliness and ways to overcome them when we are locked down.

Less Money: Feeling concerned about our money condition, housing situation, or employment situation might have a negative impact on our mental health. Money and housing: Being without a job can shake up our sense of purpose and make it challenging to keep our self-confidence intact.

Land problems: Having problems with our landlords, making repairs to our homes, or keeping up with our mortgage payments may all have an adverse effect on our mental health. Being homeless is a very traumatic experience, and it may make it much more challenging for a person whose mental health is already fragile to achieve a full recovery.

Alterations in conditions: The progression of life is unstoppable. Whether the shift is welcome or unwelcome, unexpected or foreseen, we could still find it difficult to adjust. Our mental health can be impacted by a variety of life changes, such as moving, switching schools, getting older, having a kid, starting a new career, or going to college.

Physical health: Issues with our health, such as chronic sickness, life-threatening disease, long-term illness, as well as medical visits and tests, can have a negative impact on our mental health and cause feelings of anxiety and depression in people. The most current COVID-19 epidemic is a scenario that has many individuals concerned for their own health and well-being. Visit this page to learn more about how to care for yourself and others during the outbreak of the coronavirus (COVID-19).

Addiction and substance abuse: Poor mental health can becaused by smoking, gambling, abusing drugs and alcohol, and so on. Poor mental health can, in turn, lead to increased drug abuse and behaviors characterized by addiction. This has the potential to become a never-ending loop.

Neurochemistry: The study of chemicals, such as neurotransmitters and other compounds that have an influence on the way neurons carry out their functions is referred to as neurochemistry. Neurons are nerve cells that are found in the brain and are responsible for both sending and receiving messages. Both the anatomy and the neurochemistry of the brain might leave a person open to the possibility of developing a mental disease. For instance, due to the damage that is inflicted to the brain, a person who has had a traumatic brain injury may develop mental illness as a result of their experience.

Positive Factors:

- **Experience love**

Individuals who have strong relationships with their loved ones and in which they are trusted and accepted greatly increase their odds of having a healthy self-esteem. Also, they are more likely to experience feelings of calm, safety, and confidence. They also have greater interpersonal skills and can form deeperconnections with others.

- **Self-esteem**

This is connected to how highly we think of ourselves, how well we see ourselves, and how valuable we consider ourselves to be. Those who value themselves highly are confident in theirabilities and content with who they are.

- **Confidence**

Instilling youth with self-assurance is essential to face obstacles, take chances, and develop their unique abilities. Youth who are encouraged to have faith in themselves are more likely to grow up with a healthy self-image and achieve success in all they do. This is because raising children to have confidence in themselves increases their chances of achieving their goals inlife.

- **Diet**

The mental health benefits of eating a well-balanced diet aremany. It's quite likely that it'll have profound effects on our sense of self and on our emotions on several levels, from the strictly biological to the psychological.5.

Workout. On a physiological level, studies have shown that there may be an increased risk of depression if we are deficient in certain minerals, such as iron and vitamin B12. A greater possibility of having negative feelings is linked to this risk. Our bodies are sensitive to stimulants like coffee when we are feeling particularly worried or anxious, which will heighten the feelings of worry that we are going through.

- **Building strong relationships with otherpeople**

People want connection. It is something that we need from birth. On the other hand, one does not absolutely have to be alone in order to feel lonely. Likewise, one does not have to feellonely in order to be alone. All people have a different need to feel connected to others.

Mental health, especially sadness, anxiety, and low self-esteem, may be severely impacted by long-term loneliness. In terms of mental health, loneliness is not a problem in and of itself, but the two are very closely associated, and the former cancause the latter.

Importance of Mental Well-being:

The state of one's mental health affects every person on the planet. It's likely that you know someone who has struggled with mental illness and is now on the road to recovery or who is still battling issues like anxiety, depression, addiction, or an eating disorder.

Keeping yourself healthy is crucial if you want to have a full and productive life. The development of illness can be slowed or shortened by cultivating and maintaining skills and techniques that promote healing and health. A healthy lifestyle involves more than just avoiding illness; it also involves knowing when and why to seek help and having the mental and emotional fortitude to overcome obstacles like stigma. Constructing homeostasis and well-being requires attention to one's diet, exercise, sufficient sleep, positive self- image, and the cultivation of coping skills that promote resilience. Everyone experiences stress at some point in their life, and the only way to keep one's mental health in check in the face of potentially crippling stress is to develop healthy coping techniques.

The state of being whole and sound is an essential component of wellness. Being emotionally, physically, spiritually, and mentally healthy requires balancing all of these aspects. To be willing to take care of one's mental health implies taking stock of one's moods, emotions, stress levels, and coping methods, and even being examined for various mental illnesses in the same manner that one would get screened for a variety of physical ailments. To maximize the potential for a person to enjoy a long and fruitful life, it is necessary to take a holistic approach to one's health and well-being by working to better one's mind, body, and spirit.

Wellness will also contribute to avoiding mental health issues and conditions related to drug use, as well as promoting societal aspects such as higher academic accomplishment by our children, a more productive economy, and stable family structures.

Measuring Well-being:

It is often accepted that assessing mental health is more challenging than assessing physical health or other forms of health. This is partly because there is limited availability of accurate biological testing in psychiatry, and the diagnostic criteria might vary from patient to patient. Differences in the mental health care that people receive in different parts of the world, in addition to the complexities of the social and psychological aspects, are also factors that contribute. However, in this field of research, not only is it feasible to measure the impact that the built environment has on mental health, but it is also something that is sought. Using this approach, it is feasible to show and better understand the influence that urban planning and design have on a person's mental health.

Collecting existing data:

A wide variety of study findings in the mental health field can be assessed without the need for specialized tools. The growth of big data and data related to hospital records or social media has opened the door to the use of additional markers of mental health, such as demographic information, diagnosis, police records, medication information, psychologist attendance, referrals, or health history. A person's mental health can be predicted by several factors outside their attendance at therapy sessions, such as their demographics, medical history, medicines, prescriptions, referrals, and even criminal records. Participants are often asked to self-report any psychiatric diseases they may be experiencing or medications they may be taking in place of undergoing a formal diagnostic process. This is done to improve the accuracy of the results.

It is of the utmost importance to ascertain whether or not the information that one wants is already accessible or whether or not the investment of time, effort, and focus required to gather fresh data are essential.

Biologically oriented units of measurement:

Even though there are several 'biological' tests that can be performed and are frequently utilized in the field of psychiatric research, these tests are not particularly helpful when it comes to the investigation of the majority of mental health conditions.

Interrogation for the aim of diagnosis:

A thorough psychiatric interview done by licensed professionals is the gold standard for diagnosing and determining the severity of a person's mental health issue. Most nations recognize psychiatrists and clinical psychologists as the most competent mental health professionals. These in-depth interviews take up to two hours to conduct and are used to diagnose a plethora of mental health disorders. In contrast, urban planning studies are often well-suited to assessing the impacts of environmental exposures on large populations. This is so because urban planning studies pay special attention to the built environment. Because of this, it is probably not practicable for any study project to involve psychiatrists or psychologists in the process of evaluating a very large number of people in this manner.

Methods and instruments for preliminary testing and screening:

The goal of developing screening tools for mental health is to assess specific aspects of a person's mental health with much less time and fewer resources than diagnostic interviews while still achieving nearly the same level of accuracy. This is done in response to the scale, time, and resource constraints of conducting in-depth psychiatric interviews for large populations. These screenings evaluate specific facets of an individual's mental health. These interviews are typically much shorter and are the type that almost anyone can successfully conduct after only a few hours of training. Self-administered uestionnaires are distributed to people in a specific area or who fit a certain profile; these are then either mailed back or handed directly to interviewers for processing. The information gathered from these surveys is then analyzed. This practice is quickly becoming the standard in today's world. The patient may benefit greatly from these technologies providing a continuous variable rather than a discrete clinical diagnostic.

Conclusion

People's reports of feeling content with their life have broad societal relevance since they provide insight into what matters most to them. The foundation of happiness rests on secure housing and steady employment. Policymakers need to keep an eye on these metrics. However, many metrics that assess the quality of life do not capture the quality of relationships, positive emotions, and resilience, actualizing one's potential and the overall happiness with one's existence (together referred to as "well-being"). Overall happiness and how one feels daily, from sadness to joy, is what we mean when we talk about someone's well-being.

A positive sense of self-awareness, self-respect, and self-acceptance are all components of emotional health. This paves the way for people to meet the challenges of everyday life by helping them weather the inevitable storms of health, change, and disaster. Emotional health entails identifying, honing in on, and operating from one's strengths rather than fixing problems or covering up one's weaknesses.

Emotional health does not mean never feeling sad or angry; rather, it means being in tune with your body, senses, and intuition to respond in a way that brings you into harmony withyour life's purpose.

Emotional health is boosted through people's connections with others. To thrive in society, one must learn to communicate effectively and build supportive relationships with others. One's social well-being is defined by their relationships with others and their awareness of how their actions impact the people and places around them.

It is very unusual for us to struggle with interconnection within our practices and communities since we believe we "must" be the foundation for our customers, patients, families, and communities. Many veterinarians, solo or as part of big group practices, put themselves or feel placed on their professional island, which often spills over into our personal life.

Many veterinarians are informed or believe they are "givers" or "doers," and they picked this profession as their "passion" and "calling." However, many people have never stopped to build a larger feeling of acceptance for the "person" that lies behind these labels. For many, these identities produce internal conflict when we cannot handle the demands of daily life, whether emotionally or professionally, when our "passion" does not coincide with our mission.

Whereas Physical well-being is also linked to and synergistic with social and emotional well-being. Being able to eat healthily. Hydrate. Rest well. Being proactive rather than reactive allows us to devote more attention to our mental wellness. Being preventative rather than destructive. These are the foundational aspects that build the groundwork for physical well-being. Balanced physical health will allow you to perform your everyday tasks and duties without feeling tired or stressed. We must not overlook physical fitness and all that it entails in a vocation that may shatter all of these bricks while demanding our longevity.

CHAPTER 7

MENTAL WELL-BEING

We can't separate our mental wellness from our physical health. Biological and physical aspects of wellness are typicallyprioritized in the public's mind, such as the state of our bodies, the quality of the food we consume, and the amount of activity we get. There is still something missing here in terms of health, though. The term "mental well-being" refers to the state of mind that includes our internal experiences and the words we use to express those experiences.

Six Factors Model for Mental-Being:

For one's mental well-being to be in good shape, one must persevere through the inevitable ups and downs of life and still succeed in their varied relationships, careers, hobbies, and other aspects of life. Confidence is the realization that our difficulties do not define us and the conviction that we can resolve them.

Happiness and the psychological order of humans are two different variations. How happiness and psychological functioning relate to one another and how they differ from one another are already hot topics of discussion. It is feasible to discuss "Ruff's Six" in this construct. This paradigm is used to describe psychological functioning at its best.

Carol Ryff is the author of the six-factor model of psychological well-being, a hypothesis. It establishes that six elements have a role in a person's psychological health, satisfaction, and happiness. A common query among people is: What constitutes a good life? A good life frequently has connections to well-being and a joyful, fulfilled existence. A sense of autonomy, personal growth and development, significance in life, and promising, gratifying relationships with others are all components of psychological well-being. Personal well-being is also a matter of opinion; it is generally believed that happiness and satisfaction are the two factors that determine well-being. Aristotle believed that men's pursuit of happiness was their primary motivation in ancient Greek culture. This paradigm is based on the idea that "not only the presence of something nice but also the absence of disease" is important.

Individuals rate on a scale from 1 to 6, with one indicating strongly disagreeing and six indicating strongly agreeing, with everything else falling in between, on the Ryff Scale of Measurement. Aristotle's Nicomachean Ethics, "where the objective of life isn't about feeling good but, but instead about living virtuously," is a key component of Ryff's scale and/or model.

Autonomy, personal development, environmental mastery, supportive, positive relationships, purpose in life, and self-acceptance are the six pillars upon which the Ryff Scale rests. Scores that are higher on tests are indicative of greater mental health. I've included brief explanations of each factor below.

The following is a list of Carol Ryff's six factors of well-being:

1)   Personal Growth

A high score indicates that the person is open to change and growth and that they appreciate their own and others' potential for development through time. Many people believe they are developing positively, expanding their horizons, and maturing into their full potential. Their understanding of themselves grows, and they pick up additional abilities as a bonus. Individuals scoring lower have less excitement and novelty in their lives. They appear disinterested in living, and they report feeling stagnant.

Strong Personal Growth: You have a sense of progress, growth, and expansion; you welcome new experiences; you feellike you're living up to your full potential; you observe steady, positive changes in yourself and your actions; you're becomingmore self-aware and effective as a result of these changes.

Weak Personal Growth: You feel like you've hit a mental roadblock and are unable to learn new skills or adopt other perspectives on life.

2)   Self-Acceptance

Those that score highly have a healthy perspective on their own worth as a person and the decisions they have made in the past. Participants will be asked to assess how much they accept themselves. Those that are highly accepting of themselves are comfortable with who they are and can embrace all of who they are, flaws and all. People who struggle with self-acceptance areharsh judges of their own actions and experiences. They have trouble establishing who they are and constantly want to change to become someone who is wonderful in everyone else's sight.

High Self-Acceptance: You have a healthy perspective on yourself, recognize and appreciate a variety of parts of who you are, including both your positive and negative characteristics, and have a constructive outlook on your previous lives.

Low Self-Acceptance: You are unhappy with who you are, with what has happened in your life up until this point, with specific aspects of your personality that concern you, and you have a strong desire to be someone other than who you now are.

3)   Positive Relations with Others

With a high score here, you show that you are open to change and growth, appreciate your and others' progress through time and are willing to work to make the world a better place. Many people believe they are developing and maturing constructively. Both their awareness of themselves and their capacity to learn to expand. Individuals scoring lower have less excitement and novelty in their lives. Apathy and a sense that nothing is getting better in their lives appear to be the norm these days.

Strong Positive Relations: Your interactions with others are warm, gratifying, and trustworthy; you care deeply about the people in your life; you have the capacity for deep empathy, tenderness, and closeness; and you know how to negotiate the demands and rewards of interpersonal connections.

Weak Relations: You struggle to form strong, trustworthy connections with others; you have difficulty being warm, open, and caring about others; you feel lonely and unfulfilled in your social interactions, and you refuse to make concessions to maintain your most essential friendships and relationships.

4)   Purpose in Life

Those who do well on this have a strong drive toward their goals and a firm belief that their lives serve a greater purpose. They are motivated to make a difference in the world and feel a strong bond to their ideals due to their work. These individuals know what they want out of life. People with low self-worth believe their lives are meaningless. They believe that their sole purpose in life is to finish off a few loose ends.

Strong Purpose in Life: You have a sense of direction and a set of goals for where you want your life to go, you believe that your experiences up to this point have been meaningful, and you have core values that you want to live by.

Weak Purpose in Life: You have no worldview or ideas that give life meaning, no clear sense of direction, no idea what you want out of life, and no idea what the point of your previous lives was.

5)   Environmental Masters

It indicates how much control the population has over its physical surroundings. Whether or not they believe they have the skills necessary to deal with the circumstances. A high score here indicates the individual can make good use of the resources at their disposal and is conscious of the need to control their immediate surroundings to meet their specific requirements. Those with a low score may feel helpless and unequipped to handle their surroundings. Those with low scores consistently experience high levels of anxiety and tension.

High Environmental Mastery: You are confident in your ability to shape and direct your surroundings to meet your needs and those of those you care about. You are in charge of a wide range of external activities, you make the most of the opportunities presented to you, and you select or create environments that are conducive to your goals and ideals.

Low Environmental Mastery: You have trouble keeping up with the demands of daily life, are powerless to alter or enhance contextual factors, are blind to possibilities, and feel as though you have no influence on the world at large.

6)   Autonomy

In this context, individuals are asked to assess how much control they have over. If a person scores well on this dimension, it shows that they are self-reliant and able to control their behavior without being influenced by others. They can think for themselves and exhibit independence. They don't care what other people think of them and refuse to change. Those who have a low sense of autonomy tend to rely heavily on the help of others. They care too much about what others think of them, so they try to change to fit in.

High Autonomy: You can think and act independently of others, to self-regulate your actions, and judge your worth based on your criteria.

Low Autonomy: You care what other people think of you, base major life choices on what others say, and give in to peer pressure to think and act a certain way.

Conclusion:

The framework that is provided by Carol Ryff's model of psychological well-being is an effective tool for analyzing and organizing one's life, as well as for generating ideas about how to live a better life. All of the topics covered in this chapter play a part in our everyday lives, contributing to our development as individuals. The research provides a guideline for human beings that may be adhered to impact their lives significantly.

On the other hand, although an untested model is nothing more than a pipe dream, Carol Ryff's model of psychological well-being has been subjected to several waves of testing, and the results have shown that it is surprisingly resilient. Squabbling over the questionnaires that attempt to measure the six criteria is endemic to the field of psychology and is a common practice in the field. In spite of this, researchers that worked with samples from a wide variety of populations discovered that the findings are consistent with and can be described most well by a model composed of six factors.

Some data contradicts itself, arguing that the six criteria may be reduced because considerable overlaps have been observed in their application. Ryff contends that these conflicting findings were due to too short surveys rather than the model itself, despite the fact that other research has failed to detect the overlap of this nature.

CHAPTER 8

STEP TOWARDS IMPROVEMENT

Have you ever noticed how everything seems manageable when you're in a good mood?

Or how a problem doesn't seem so serious after you've woken up from a good rest? Or how a phone call to a friend makes you feel so much better?

The effects of our mental health are experienced in every aspect of our lives. Our moods, physical health, and social connections help us cope better with adversity and unexpected hurdles. Together, they contribute to our sense of well-being and our mental health. By taking a proactive stance of improving, maintaining, and nurturing our mental health, we can ensure that we live healthy, productive, and meaningful lives.

What can positive mental health look like? Here are two examples:

• Brenda is a stay-at-home mom. Now that her children have moved out, she has more leisure time. She has started studying a new language and attends community college. Despite being an older student, she likes her studies and works hard. Her professors' opinions and her colleagues' relationships enhance her sense of meaning and purpose.

- Jones is late for his meeting. Instead of belittling himself for just being late, he reminds himself that he has no control over all of life's circumstances. Out of courtesy to the rest of the office, he gives them 15 minutes' notice. He doesn't think of his procrastination as a flaw in his personality, and he promises never to be late again.

Importance of Mental Well-being

Good mental well-being involves two things: feeling good and functioning well. You experience happiness, optimism, compassion, satisfaction, and contentment in your emotions, have a sense of purpose, and develop positive relationships.

Physical and mental health are not thought of as separate things because good physical health can lead to better mental health, leading to a better life, and the other way around.

Having good mental health doesn't just affect how you appear. It also shapes the way and how you act. Your mental health condition can also impact your workplace performance, which in turn affects society. For example, people who work in stressful jobs can get burned out. As a result, they are less likely to enjoy their jobs and can get sick.

To avoid or reduce the severity of certain mental illnesses and disorders, people might want to pay more attention to their own mental health in a constructive way. This could also help them in other areas of life, such as one's physical health and work life.

It's almost too easy to ignore the importance of taking care of our mental health in pursuit of more pressing matters. It's also possible that you'll think it's too huge and difficult to handle. It's not, however.

Happiness, resilience, and self-confidence are all part of our new definition of mental health and well-being. The following is a list of mental well-being advantages based on this comprehensive approach.

•   Positive outcomes, such as positive connections, higher revenue, ability to cope with stress, and longer life expectancy, are connected to a person's level of happiness.

•   As a result of enhanced mental health, people are more inclined to engage in physical activity.

•   The ability to fulfill one's goals is enhanced when experiencing a sense of improved well-being.

•   Positive emotions allow people to meet new people and increase their resources for future adversity.

•   Anger and irritation can be reduced by engaging in activities that make you happy, such as gardening or flower-growing, going for walks outside, or spending time with animals.

•   A better sense of well-being can encourage relaxation in your life. A mental break from these sensations might help you refocus and get your mind back in the game.

Factors That Can Influence YourMental Well-Being

The situational factors are external interventions that can affect the lives of young children to older adults. Several situational conditions may put some teenagers at a higher risk ofsocial, sentimental, and mental well-being problems.

All individuals fear, stress, or depression due to certain events in their lives. A variety of variables in life might influence your psychological health. These elements can either jeopardize or safeguard your mental health.

All are unique, and we all exist under unique situations. Risk and protective variables are also unique to each individual and alter through time, such as a child, adolescent, adult, or older person.

You may enhance your mental health and wellness by increasing the protective elements in your life and decreasing therisk factors.

Let's talk about some of the situational factors that can actually dent one's mental health.

Bullying

Bullying may strike anybody, at any time, and in any place. It can occur in classrooms, at homes, at the workplace, in internet community places, through SMS, or through the mail. Bullying is defined as a persistent abuse of power in relationships that results in bodily or psychological injury through repeated verbal, physical, or social behavior. It might entail a single person or a group abusing their authority over one or many people. Bullying can occur in public settings, and it canbe pervasive or insidious.

In any form or context, bullying may have long-term consequences for everyone engaged, including bystanders.

Individual incidences, disputes, or arguments among peers, whether online or in person, are not considered bullying.

Isolation

Most people suffer feelings of isolation or solitude at some point. These sensations are natural and typically dissipate, but ifthey do not pass and continue for an extended period of time, they can negatively influence your psychological health and welfare. People have felt disconnected for a variety of reasons. Some of the causes might be: emotions of loss or sadness, mental health concerns or illnesses due to poor physical health or frailty(e.g., depression, anxiety) and a loss of meaning or purpose in life, linguistic hurdles, or fewer links with your culture.

Unemployment

Joblessness, layoff, company failure, big investment losses, or other negative externality can all negatively influence your mental health. Taking care of your mental health and well-beingwill help you deal with the stress and concern of getting laid offor losing a business. You can take easy and practical things to maintain your mental health and well-being throughout this period.

Keeping a usual consistent schedule may bring numerous benefits, including a sense of better control over your life and a common purpose, and help you focus on essential things. It also helps you schedule time in your day to take care of your mentalhealth and well-being.

Drug and Alcohol Abuse

People going through a challenging time in their lives may resort to substance misuse to help them deal. There is a clear association between the use of alcohol and other drugs and mental health problems.

Alcohol and other substances can be used to relieve those who are suffering from mental health concerns. Alcohol and substance use can also trigger anxiety, despair, psychosis, and hallucinations in persons predisposed to mental health problems.

The use of alcohol and other drugs alters how you behave, feel, and make decisions. While somebody might use alcohol or other substances because they believe they will make them feel better in the short term, they can really make you feel worse in the long run, particularly if you have a mental health condition.

Insomnia

A restful night's sleep is critical to our personal health and well-being. Sleep deprivation may have a significant influence on our mood, attention, memory, and overall quality of life. 29.

The quantity of 'deep sleep' a person obtains, rather than the length of sleep, determines good quality sleep.

Everyone has difficulty sleeping from time to time. This might involve having difficulty falling asleep or waking up regularly and being unable to return to sleep.

How Can People Around You Ruin Your Mental Health?

There are several reasons for mental health disorders. Many

people are likely to be touched by a complex combination of circumstances, while various persons may be more profoundly affected by specific things than others.

Although job, nutrition, medicines, and sleep deprivation can all have an influence on human health, if you have a mental health problem, there are generally additional elements at play.

After all, we are mortal. When people are unable to connect with us and interact in a healthy manner, we might feel unwanted, unwelcome, or as if we don't belong. It's difficult not to accept your disconnection as a judgment on your own value. How can you not listen to what others have to say?

We've all had somebody say rude things to us at some point in our lives. They can sometimes longer be with us or eventually wind up with us retaining the sensations we are left with. Words may be hurtful. They can exacerbate clinical depression unless you're already susceptible to it, and they might leave you feeling irritated, rejected, ashamed, discouraged, or simply unhappy.

How to Recognize Toxicity around You?

You may be dealing with a toxic person if you know

someonewho is tough and generates a lot of friction in your life. These people may cause a great deal of tension and discomfort for you and others, not to mention mental or even bodily suffering.

A toxic person is someone whose attitude causes you to be unhappy. People that are toxic are frequently struggling with their own anxieties and traumas. To accomplish this, they behave in ways that do not put them in a better light andfrequently irritate others in the process.

Toxicity is not considered a disability in humans. However, there might be inherent psychological illness causing someone to act in harmful ways, such as a narcissistic personality.

So here are a few red flags to look out for if you suspect you're working with a toxic person:

- You have the impression that you are beingcoerced into doing something you do not want to do.
- You're continuously perplexed by the person's actions.
- You believe you are entitled to an apology, but it never arrives.

- You must always protect yourself.
- You're never really at ease with them.
- In their presence, you constantly feel horrible about yourself.

Mental Abuse

There are a variety of ways to mistreat or abuse someone's emotional well-being. You may not see it until it's too late. It might come in waves of perfect quiet, or it can arrive at any time.

You may not realize whether you're being emotionally abused until it's too late. A few indications may be unnoticed byyou. It's possible you've been told you're hyper-emotional or thatthis is how all relationships are.

It's important to pay notice if you start to feel alone, helpless, or useless in your relationships. There is no justification for youto feel this way. All of these things are rightfully yours.

Let's first talk about what mental abuse is.

Threats, taunts, and other insidious methods of mind manipulation are all manifestations of mental abuse. This type of abuse is particularly distressing since it is clearly intended todamage a person's feeling of self-worth and self-confidence, as well as their perception of reality or their own abilities.

Mental abuse is a kind of 'mental brutality' and 'intimate terrorism' because of the serious consequences of this behavior. Gaslighting is a prevalent kind of psychological abuse in whichone person is made to believe that they are crazy. This is when an abuser may distort the facts, causing a person to distrust theirown recollections and perceptions.

In some cases, an event that occurred in the summer may be modified to take place in the winter, or possibly not at all. Reactionary conduct is common when the individual being manipulated attempts to resist or fight back against the manipulation. As a result of their feelings of helplessness and frustration, their responses are impulsive and unpredictable. When an abuser does this, they are eroding their own self-esteemas well as the respect of others around them.

Psychiatric abuse focuses on methods of shame, insult, fear, or exploitation. Finally, reality and one's self-worth are related to an abusive individual.

- **Signs to Notice**

If you notice some or all of these attitudes and behaviors, it signals the fact that the person is emotionally abusing you. These include:

- **Name-Calling**

Abusers often resort to using abusive language as a way to degrade and belittle their victims. Even small infractions, such as forgetting to take out the garbage or mispronouncing a foreign phrase, are sufficient to denigrate or humiliate someone.

- **Blaming**

When someone is emotionally abusing you, they may "turn the switch," blaming you for the actions or responses of others. When someone says, "I wouldn't have done that if you hadn't gotten me so upset," they're blaming someone else for their own actions.

- **Accusing**

People-pleasing attitudes can be triggered by false allegations. It's possible to go to great efforts to be attentive to someone who is accusing you of cheating. Additionally, you may avoid leaving the house for fear of a confrontation with your family members over your whereabouts.

- **Making Threats**

Threats are a popular trick used by those who exploit another person's mind, whether it's to destroy a relationship or take away your children. To keep someone in a permanent state of horror or fear, threats can be used. A mismatch in power is generated by intimidation. Putting the other under their thumb offers one individual an advantage over the other.

- **Neglecting**

When a person's bodily or mental needs are unmet, this can be interpreted as neglect. Emotional neglect can take the form of withholding love or punishing and abusing you silently.

What can you do when you're mentally abused, and it's becoming so toxic that you can't even breathe?

If your relationship experiences the signs and repercussions of mental abuse, obtaining therapy while you are still safe has to be a priority.

This is not always simple. Reaching out for support might be frightening to contemplate. Not simply to avoid the notion of your abuser discovering it, but also because sharing what you'vebeen through might be difficult.

This may be embarrassing or a cause of shame for anyone. It may be more challenging to get treatment if you are in a position of prestige or are on a high-achiever path at work or in other social circles. You remain mute among those who can assist you out of fear of losing your identity and standing within that group. That loss may seem excessive in exchange for an uncertain outcome.

However, mental abuse can result in significant harm. This risk is always greater if you are constantly exposed to abuse. The good news is that having a workplace to go to may provide a sense of security and confidence. The disadvantage is that you are carrying a considerable amount of unnecessary stress and issues that your manager or supervisor is absolutely ignorant of
- attempting to maintain two separate lives may be incredibly tough.

How to Leave a Toxic Situation?

A black hole is filling you with anger and frustration, and

youcan't get out. There doesn't seem to be a way out of this dilemma of bad energy and thoughts, no matter how hard you try to get out of it. There is nothing that you feel you can do to get better after these emotions.

As you can see, these are the feelings and mood disturbances we have when we are stuck in terrible situations in our lives.

Most of us will feel this way at some point in our lives, whether it's about our professional or personal life. The effect is bad on all edges and can cause a lot of depressive episodes, no matter what.

However, this is not a problem that can't be addressed. With the right approach and attitude, we can not only fight this miserybut also use it to accomplish something great in our lives.

You can develop personal traits to cater to mental health problems by ignoring people. Here are some of the things you can do to get rid of the toxicity in your life.

Don't Take It Personal

It is often not about what someone speaks to us, but about themselves. They may be unhappy or dissatisfied with themselves and may strike out at others to feel better. It's possible that they're having a horrible day. You may also need to give the other individual the due credit. Whatever the reason for someone saying anything that may have a bad impact on you, you do not have to take it to heart.

Take Lessons

It takes work to learn how to absorb remarks or criticism constructively rather than hurtfully. We are always "becoming." It's acceptable if you don't answer every comment flawlessly or do everything exactly—even if you think you could. That is something to aim for at all times. Take some time to ponder any comments or criticism directed at you if they are true. Even if it wasn't expressed in the best way, check if there's anything you can do better for yourself so you may have a happier life.

Change Your Perception

If someone repeatedly criticizes you, it's more than just trying not to take it personally and letting them go.

You will begin to perceive things through a modern perspective as you practice new approaches. This will therefore enable you to have better connections with others, particularly with yourself. It takes time, as well as regular awareness and effort, to not be affected by what people say. Your objective is to discover hope, happiness, and tranquility in order to improve your mental health.

Analyze Your Circumstances

Study all sides of the problem to figure out what is going on. How can you make things better for yourself and for the people around you? After you figure out what caused the situation, you can start taking steps to get out of it. Do not put off this, no matter how hard critical reflection might be.

Set Your Limits

People who are toxic don't do well with rules. They have a strong desire to want to be in charge of other people and situations. If you try to set limits or boundaries for them, you won't get anywhere. They see it as a personal challenge.

The thing is, though, that there are limits to how much power you can have over certain things. Don't spend too much time or exertion with people who are bad for you. Conversations should be short, and the topics should be light, too. Those who aren't good for you should keep in mind that they'll be listening for anything you say that they can twist, so they look better.

So, talk about the weather, or say nice things about somebody. And then you run away from that person as fast as you can. Use your phone's timer if you need to. Take the old SOS route from somebody you trust. Do what you need to do to get out of this situation.

Focus on the Positive

Well yeah, it is a cliché, but if you think about how annoying toxic people can be or the problems they make, it will make you stressed to the point of not being able to do anything.

Do your best to acknowledge when you begin to focus on the negativity and try to think of solutions or better situations instead. People who are bad for you don't deserve your mental power.

Limit Your Social Media Interactions

Try to cut down on how much time you spend talking to toxic people on the internet. Staying close to a friend who makes you jealous, posts things that make you angry, or talks bad about you can have a big impact on your mental and emotional health.

What's worse, your friend's actions and statements aren't theonly wrong things. The Internet, especially social media, is a seemingly endless source of antagonistic interactions among people.

Remember That Recovery Is a Long Process

If you don't see immediate changes, don't be angry at yourself for not seeing them right away. Think about how long it will take to get rid of your depression and other bad habits. There is a better chance that you will move in the right direction if you work hard at small changes and celebrate your small victories asyou go.

CHAPTER 9

PERSONAL WELL-BEING

So far, we've discussed what physical and mental health are, their importance, types, and what affects these aspects of your life. This last part of the book mainly focuses on the personal factors that contribute to your mental health. These can include your mindset, relationships, mental health problems, and perspective on life.

Mental health issues can often result from social isolation, long-term stress, physical health condition, childhood abuse, and neglect. But apart from that, your present life and how you view yourself as a person can greatly impact your mental health.

Putting Yourself First

Create a mindset of putting yourself first. We know what you may be thinking: *but it's selfish to think about yourself before others*. Let's burst this little bubble of yours. It's not selfish. Loving yourself before you start to love others is critical to seeking fulfillment and happiness in life.

If you want to live a life where your needs are met, you feel good about yourself and start caring for yourself. It may seem difficult at first, but eventually, this pathway can lead to better relationships, high performance at work, and inner satisfaction. If half your cup is full, it's easier to be a giver than with a half cup empty. Right? That's how you can change your perspective and fulfill your needs first to preserve more for others.

Rules may change, and they may not always be the same. What might work once in your life might not the next time. It doesn't mean that you can't get through things with a positive mind. You just have to take a different approach. Your past or your present may distract you from this path. It can be unsent messages, pressures of life, tragedies, and societal influences. You can get confused, and that's okay. Your mind may trick you into believing the negative, but it will pass.

You need to understand that life is not always easy, but you need to be constant throughout it. It can come with many sacrifices but your motivation to do something should stem from meaningfulness.

You can't carry passengers if you don't fill your gas tank. You can't help others if you don't put your oxygen mask on.

The best and the worst part of being a human is that you can't always be there for everyone and not everyone can save you. Carve out moments of peace for yourself and change your life because you can do that. You can work on yourself.

Consider your feelings because no one else is going to. Maybe yes, your mother, but even then, she's a human with a body and soul too. Here are some of the ways in which you can prioritize yourself without causing anyone hurt.

Small Ways to Put Yourself First

- Set Boundaries with People

Learn to say no to things you don't want to do. Boundaries are the best way to tell others what you're okay with, what you don't want, or how you don't want to be treated. You can also set your boundaries about sharing personal information, understanding personal needs, valuing opinions, or accepting when others say no. Be assertive and safeguard your space!

- Do Something That Makes You Happy

This provides your mind a break from doing the same thing over and over again. In today's world, it seems as though we are always working. But there needs to be a balance in life. Do something you enjoy in order to neutralize the stress. This is a nice relief from the daily grind.

- Take Time Out for Yourself

Smile at yourself in the mirror. It may spread like wildfire. Haven't you heard? Smile is contagious. It boosts your mood and those around you. The best part about smiling even when no one is there is that you don't need someone to smile back at you. Your brain automatically interprets your smile as a sign of joy. It's a quick method that has a big impact on your life.

- Set Alarms

There is no need to stress about waking up at 5am every day, but getting into an organized habit will help you make time for yourself every day. It's a little gesture that serves as a daily reminder to embrace self-care, whether it's waking up 20 minutes earlier each day or setting the alarm to remind you to work out or meditate.

- Develop a Self-Care Practice

Maintain a pattern of self-care. Many of us fall short in this area. Perhaps once in a while, we'll remember to do these things. However, if you truly want to make yourself a priority, you need to make this a regular routine. Morning and nighttime rituals have been proven to be some of the most effective approaches to promoting self-care sustainability. The primary advantage of having a morning routine is that it gives you time to tend to your needs before the day's events arise. It's also a great way to start your day off on the right foot. A nighttime ritual, on the other hand, can help you wind down after a long day and get ready for bed.

- Take a Break from Social Media

We don't spend enough time with ourselves. Constantly, it's either an Instagram notification, a WhatsApp message, or a PUBG match that takes you to the screen world. You need to take a break at least once an hour. Unplug all your devices, keep them aside, and focus on where your mind wanders.

Social media is often argued to be one of the reasons you feel negative and insecure about yourself, and we agree with that. It puts pressure on you and makes you feel bad about yourself. Take some time out and enjoy the real-life experiences in front of you.

- Invest in Relationships with People Who Put YouFirst

Keep yourself in the company of individuals who inspire and motivate you. Spending time with people who don't get along with you might drain your energy. Also, our brains may be easily manipulated. Being around negative people who don't encourage you, you may suffer the same consequences. At times, it grows to be too much and becomes exhausting. So, surround yourself with those who shine a spotlight and offer joyful vibes. Because this is a fun way to be accompanied.

Putting yourself first ensures that you don't end up sucking the joy out of your life. If you know your habits and still, you don't encourage yourself to change them, it can sabotage your mental health.

Self-Sabotaging Behaviors That Are Ruining YourRelationships

Sabotaging, in easy words, means destroying or perhaps crippling your relationships with those you care about or who care about you. Your mental health has a strong link with your relationships and connections. If you're happily married or have a stable relationship, it may positively impact your mental healthand lower stress and depression.

Relationships may have ups and downs, but how do you or your partner treat these speed breakers? Are you sabotaging your relationship, or do you fear that your partner is determined to end it with you?

Let's talk about both perspectives here.

You met someone new a few months back, and the chemistry is strong, and the sex is fun. Then, you spend more and more time together and start talking about moving in or committing tobecoming a serious couple.

But then, all of a sudden, one of you stops replying to texts, there are no more calls, and the dates are being canceled. You avoid sharing everything, and anger, frustration, and disappointment come into the picture. This may be breaking your relationship.

If this sounds like something that has happened with you or is happening, you're sabotaging your relationship.

There can be several reasons why you or your partner may be sabotaging your relationship. It can be anything from first relationship experience to parenting and childhood. Your past experiences and your present thoughts can all have an impact onhow you act today.

Defensiveness, affairs, partner harassment, destructive behaviors like excessive gambling, contempt, partner withdrawal, trusting difficulty, and jealousy are all some ways you can sabotage your relationships. Some of the examples of self-sabotaging behaviors can include:

- Constant insecurity about your relationship.

- Making 20 calls a day just to get over your insecurity.

- The incapability of settling differences.

- Developing a victim mentality, pointing fingersat your partner.

- Texting anxiety if your partner doesn't reply immediately.

- Indulging in self-defeating thoughts andquestioning your abilities.

- Holding excessive grudges against your partner.

- Getting into alcohol abuse and addiction as a result of relationship stress.

All of these behaviors that put pressure on your relationship have a lasting impact on your mental health. It can cause stress, depression, and anxiety, making you unable to focus on your life, yourself, your professional life, and other important people in your life.

Avoid getting hurt in this process and implement different techniques in your life to respond to destructive behaviors and protect yourself or your partner. If it's your mistake, rectify it. If it's their mistake, make them acknowledge it with care and love. It can change, improvise, and your relationship can be better.

It seems easy to say this, but it takes more than just words. Here are a few ways you can stop self-sabotaging your relationships and getting mentally hurt as a result.

- **Encourage Open Communication**. It can help clear up misunderstandings and manage your expectations from your partner better.

- **Accept Things Happen**: Even in a relationship when both partners are doing their best, there may be times when one of them will feel upset, even if both seem to be doing their utmost.

• **Be Patient**: It takes a lot of patience to work on a relationship, especially when you're putting in so much effort. Be proud of yourself for identifying harmful behavior and taking the necessary steps to resolve it.

• **View Your Relationship as a Partnership**: In a committed relationship, it helps to consider your relationship as a co-creating life, and this attitude can make you excited about building a future together.

• **Don't Invest in Relationships That You Know Are Hopeless**: Having partners who are simply unsuitable for you is one way to cause romantic self- harm. Pursuing any romantic opportunity that comes your way, seek partnerships that have a chance of succeeding.

You can also consider therapy if you think that your mental health is becoming worse. If you think you're in a relationship but not ready for the long-term, a therapist can help you process the issues and shed light on something serious. There's a chance that you love your partner, but that one trait of either of you is causing all the trouble.

Changing a few habits to cope with triggers and problems is not always a bad choice. In fact, it ends up making it easier for you. A better, happier, satisfying relationship leads to a mood boost and good overall mental well-being.

How Mental Turmoil Can Harm You Physically

Poor mental health and a tired mind can lead to harmful behaviors and poor physical health. Depression can lead to chronic diseases like asthma, cancer, diabetes, and arthritis. Sleep disorders like insomnia and sleep apnea can lead to breathing problems. Smoking to relieve stress can result in lungproblems and addiction.

As they say, if you remain positive, you're more likely to have a better day. What you do and think can impact your mood and have a lasting effect on your mental well-being. One's intrinsic and learned behaviors to deal with emotions and regulate in daily life are known as *emotional intelligence*. On theother hand, engaging in social activities, taking responsibility, and valuing other people's perspectives come under the headingof *social intelligence*.

If you develop the ability to understand your intelligence levels, you're better at recognizing your behaviors, impulses, moods, and how you can best manage them. Be aware of your own emotions and others to effectively manage challenging situations and phases in life.

Change Begins on The Inside

When we discuss personal change, we address internal factors. The stupid beliefs we possess, the positive ideologies webury, and the perspectives we must develop.

Extreme changes, such as attaining our ideal weight, relocating to a new place, taking on a new profession, or entirelyupending what we consider 'normal,' do not always result in thedesired internal change.

We take along our established beliefs, anxieties, views, triggers, and attitudes wherever we go. Our external selves and circumstances may change, but our inner selves generally do not. Because when the shift we feel does not originate from inside, its consequences will be just temporary - not permanent.

YOU ARE IMPORTANT!!!

It's not selfish to put one's own well-being ahead of one's commitments. Because if you don't keep hold of yourself, how can you show concern for others? Put your own needs ahead of others for the simple reason that you have meaning and importance in this world. Every day, do three activities benefit your mind, body, and spirit.

We challenge our readers to make a commitment. Stop what you're doing and think about when the last time you put yourself first before others.

Been a while, right? Well, take a deep breath and think of how things would be different if you put yourself first. What can change? Will your relationships improve? Will you be able to achieve your goals and dreams? Will you have more time for yourself?

That's the perspective that is often lost in our busy and hectic lives.

CHAPTER 10

AN INTRODUCTION TO EMOTIONAL WELL-BEING

Emotional wellbeing is basically the ability to successfully handle the difficult times and life stress, without any difficulties. It is something that It gives us confidence to adapt to change and manage our emotions even in the times when it is the most difficult to do so. Though there are many different explanations of emotional wellbeing that are found in different books but the one that is the most relevant is that the well-being refers to the understanding and awareness we have about our emotions ad how well we are able to handle complex situations around us.

Even if we don't give our emotional wellbeing as much attention as we should but still it is very important to understand that it is something that can affect our day to day operations. If we don't keep our emotional health in check, then ultimately, we would have to suffer in some way. I must say that difficulties in emotional well-being can surely have a negative impact on our physical or mental health.

People who are emotionally healthy often have control over

their thoughts, feelings, and behavior and are able to deal with life's obstacles and overcome disappointments. Being emotionally balanced doesn't mean we never experience sadness, rage, or frustration.

Fostering resiliency, self-awareness, and a general sense of well-being require excellent emotional health. The way we receive and respond to criticism and feedback, how we offer advice, and how we observe and interpret what other people are doing and why also depend on how well we are emotionally balanced.

If we want to prosper and thrive in both our professional and personal life, we must have the abilities to maintain excellent emotional health.

For instance, as we have all observed over the past several years, the workplace is less predictable than ever before, making it more crucial than ever for us to be able to control our emotions and how we react in stressful situations

Our capacity to have the tools in place to manage both our good and negative emotions is crucial since we will inevitably confront problems in our personal life.

Signs of Emotional Wellbeing

It is very easy to tell if someone is doing emotionally well or not. Those who have a better emotional health usually look relaxed and present in the moment rather than lost in some otherthoughts. However, there are a few signs that can tell you if youare doing well emotionally or not.

- **You Are Able to Switch Off and Unwind**

The very first sign of emotionally people is that they can easily switch off the distractions around them and can unwind for some time. This means that they have the ability to block outthe thoughts that have been taking a toll on then and investing that energy in their own wellbeing these are the kind of people who know when their physical, emotion and mental self requiresa recharge.

- **You Enjoy the Present Time**

Another sign of being emotionally well is that you enjoy themoments that you are living currently. You don't regret the things that have happened in the past and either are you worriedabout the things that will come your way in future. So, if you want you are one those who live one day at a time then definitely you are doing well emotionally. Also, it is something that brings more focus and joy to your life.

- **You Sleep Soundly**

The third and the most important sign of wellbeing is that you have a sound sleep whenever you get to bed. It is not very much difficult for you to relax by packing away all your worries and everyday tasks. It has been said that the best sleeper in this world are those who don't even have to think about falling asleep; they just do it. The best sleepers are people who don't even think about falling asleep: they just do it. Moreover, it is important to understand that having a good sleep is not only helpful for emotional wellbeing but it also makes the person fresh to perform well the next day.

- **You Have A Meaning in Life**

If you know what you want from your life and you are aware that you are here for a reason then surely you are the right tract emotionally. Those people who question their existence and are mostly thinking about their motive to be in this world have a comparatively week emotional health. They don't enjoy the good things in their life and are only stuck in their thoughts of worthlessness and melancholy.

- ## You Let Resentments Go

Another sign of being emotionally strong is that you don't hold grudges against people. No matter how bad you have been treated or how awful you felt at that moment, still you let all the resentment go. This means that if someone has done something wrong to you and you are an emotionally well individual then you will have enough courage to let it go and not let it dominate you. Also, you won't let that person, place or thing live "rent free" in your head.

- ## You Take Pride in Your Appearance and Personal Hygiene

Any human who is emotionally well will definitely take care himself. He will dress up nicely and will make all possible efforts to look presentable all the time. For this they will push themselves every day to get out of bed and work out, in order to stay in shape. It is only because they value themselves and also their time – and see what they can give to the world each day. So, if you feel and react in somewhat similar way then it is a sign of emotional wellbeing.

- ### You Are Comfortable in Your Skin

Another sign of being emotionally well is that you are comfortable in your own skin. This means that you are content with how you look, what you think, also what you do and you don't seek approval from others. You feel extremely confident in front of other people and nothing really stops you from being yourself. Also, you will be courageous and confident enough to say "NO" to the things that cross your healthy boundaries.

- ### You Are Optimistic and Hopeful

Being optimistic and hopeful is also a very important sig of being emotionally well. Those who are emotionally healthy, always focus on the positives and abundance. Even if something happens against their plan or will, still they make peace with it and find something optimistic out of it. They will be full of hope and this thing will always motivate them. So, if you feel the same way then you are also among the list of people with emotional wellbeing.

- ### You Feel Connected

If you mostly feel disconnected with the world, then it is considered a key aspect of addiction. And the only solution to be addiction free is that you try to connect with the people around you and also maintain a friendly relationship. However, if you accept everyone the way they are and develop a relationship accordingly then you are said to be an emotionally sound individual.

- **You Will Have Empathy**

Well, empathy is a trait that is very hard to find these days. But, those who have strong emotional health show their genuine concern towards others and actually want to do something for them. They actively look out for people who might need help and once they find such people they go out of their way to help them. Even if they disagree with someone still they have the capability to see things from the perspective of other people. So, if you fit in this criterion then you are also emotionally sound and strong.

Factors Affecting Our EmotionalWellbeing:

If you look precisely then you will be able to find thousands of factors that affect a human's emotional wellbeing. There would be thousands of things that contribute in making a person emotionally healthy or drained. However, I have discussed some of the common ones below.

- **Physical Well-Being**

Your emotional wellbeing is somewhat related to your physical wellbeing. If you will feel fit physically and you will feel healthy from within then there are higher chances of you to feel good emotional. But, if something is not right in your physical health then it will be shown in your emotional attitude. For example, a person who is active all the time and has a healthy lifestyle is more likely to have a better emotional health that the one who feels lethargic and drained all the time. This brings to the point that, how you feel about your body and your inner self, it is reflected in your behavior. So, one must watch after his physical wellbeing if it is his goal to achieve emotional wellbeing.

- **Financial Well-Being**

Another factor that plays a very important role in your emotional and mental sanity is your financial wellbeing. With financial wellbeing I mean that you are able to earn a sufficient amount of money that helps you pay off your bills and also take care of other expenses. So, if you are doing fine financially then there will be no threat to your emotional health. But if due to any reason your earnings are not able to cover your expenses, then your emotional health will be at risk.

Those who don't have their finances sorted, often end up being addicted to alcohol or other dangerous drugs, in order to distract themselves from the thoughts of their financial problems. However, this ultimately leads to more physical and mental health issues then cannot be catered if it gets too late. So, you must keep your expenses in check and sped in accordance to what you earn, because if you go overboard (even slightly) it will start taking a toll on your mental health.

- **Career Well-Being**

Career Wellbeing is basically how you manage your career both today and also tomorrow, so that you are provided with resources, opportunities and motivation to achieve the goals you have defined for yourself. So, it would not be wrong to say that career wellbeing is simply more than the job you are in today.

Doing a job that we love and enjoy can provide us a meaning focus in life and can also fulfill our need to bring some income home. It is totally dependent on the money we make that what living standard we will be having and this is something contributes or our self-esteem and self-image. So, technically work-related issues can affect both our emotional as well as mental health. Therefore, it is necessary to keep a check on it right from the beginning.

- ### Social Well-Being

The sharing, creating, and maintaining of meaningful relationships with people can be characterized as social well- being. This gives you a sense of connection and belonging while enabling you to feel genuine and cherished.so, this gives an understanding that those who are able to maintain a positive relationship with people around them are more likely to have a better emotional health as compared to those who keep themselves isolated from the world.

Generally, it has been seen that those people who don't havefamilies to look after them or don't have friends to hand out with often suffer emotionally. It becomes difficult for them to handle their everyday tasks in the most efficient manner. In fact, getting out of bed itself is a huge task for them.

This brings me to the point that all physical, emotional, and social well-being are interlinked. Even if one thing is not doing well the other two will automatically get disrupted. For example, a person who is perfectly fine physically and also takes care of his diet has a problem with interacting with people. He finds it very difficult to interact with people even if he knows them. Eventually with time, this problem of his leaves him isolated and he starts spending most of his time alone, in his own space. Now, even if he was doing fine physically, but because of his social anxiety both his emotional as well as physical wellbeing will suffer. He might start losing weight because of his emotional instability or may also, adopt some unhealthy eating habits to deal with his anxiety.

Causes of Emotional Wellbeing

Though emotional wellbeing can be achieved through many different things but I have discussed the most important ones below to give a clear understanding.

• **Being Mindful**

The first thing that leads to emotional wellbeing is practicing mindfulness. If you will stay in the present and will try to make the most of it then will help you become more aware of the things that are going on inside you and also your surroundings. However, those who are mindful most of the time usuallyperform the following activities:

• They breathe deeply. This means that they inhale from their nose for about four seconds and they hold it in for one second. After that they exhale it through their mouth in the next five seconds. This is a part of their everyday routine and they repeat it when they find it necessary.

• They go out for walks. However, while walking they pay attention to their breathing cycle and also engage all their senses with the surrounding. Also, even if anything crosses their mind, hey just get rid of it by focusing on the good things in their life.

• They eat mindfully. By this I mean that they don't just start eating their food right away but they takeenough time to smell it and show their gratitude. After that they notice the flavors and texture of the food the food they are eating, with every single bite. Moreover, whenever their stomach gives the signal of being emptyor full, they pay attention to it.

• Lastly, they mentally scan each part of their body, from head to toe to be aware how every part of their body actually feels.

- **Managed and Reduced Stress**

Another thing that can be counted as a cause of emotional wellbeing is managed and reduced stress. When the stress is reduced or somewhat eliminated from life, a persona feels emotionally healthy. Though stress can be helpful to someextend and it might also help to get done with the tasks, but long- term stress can be awfully unhealthy. However, those who wantto achieve emotional wellbeing by reducing their stress often carry out the following activities:

- They fix their sleep schedule and try to get morethan 7 hours of sleep every night.

- They incorporate exercise and workout in their everyday routine. No matter how tough it is for them to get out of bed still they push themselves to do it every day.

- They create a positive social support network for themselves. This means that they surround themselves with people who have positive mindset so that even if they get a bit distracted, there are some people to put them back on track.

- They set boundaries and schedule their time to relax. They don't let people disturb them on the times when they don't want any invasion. However, they knowtheir priorities and they work accordingly.

•   They focus on the things that they have achieved and not on those they have lost. They make themselves feel good about all the good things they have done in lifeand whatever has brought them happiness.

•   **Having A Positive Mindset**

One of the most come cause of achieving emotional wellbeing is having a positive mindset. Those who hold onto positive emotions for longer in their life and appreciate the goodthings around them, face no issues when it comes to being emotionally strong. Those who have achieved emotional wellbeing through their positive attitude, often have the following habits

•   They recognize all the good deeds they have donefor other people.

•   They forgive themselves for all the mistakes theyhave made in the past, rather than crying over them. In fact, they make all the possible efforts to never make those mistakes later in their life.

•   They have a gratitude journal, I which they

write the things they are grateful for every day. For example, if someone is grateful for the stranger who held a door for them, then they will write about it in their journal. Though it is very small thing but it will have a very positive impact on the brain.

• They spend time with people who have a positive attitude towards life. They surround themselves with those people who take about ideas and goals, rather thanthose who only gossip and pull others down.

• Lastly, these people take very good care of their mental and physical health. They make healthy changes to their lifestyle so that they feel good about themselvesand have a positive attitude towards life.

• **Reinforced Social Connections**

Those individuals who have an emotional being usually reinforce healthy social connections. However, it is because of these connections that they are able to life an emotionally sound life.so, to create a positive support system, people adopt thefollowing behaviors:

• They join several groups that focus on interestingactivities and hobbies.

- They create a very positive relationship with their friends, family member and also children. They try to beavailable for them whenever they are in need.

- They don't shy away when it comes to asking for help from other. This means that they are emotionally very strong and they their self-confidence is also in the right place.

- They have a learning attitude. They are always looking out for different skills and activities that they canlearn.

- They volunteer in for different causes. This tells that those who are emotionally healthy often want to spread happiness around them. They can't see people suffering or going through a difficult time, so this is why they want to step in and help them in any way they could.

- They love to travel to different places and meet people belonging to different backgrounds.

CHAPTER 11

RISK BEHAVIOR

Risk Behavior is an activity that increases the probability of a person suffering from a specific condition. For example, if a person deliberately lands himself in a situation, where he knows that he might suffer then this is called risky behavior. In other words, this behavior can be defined as conscious or unconsciously controlled conduct that is accompanied by a perceived lack of assurance about the outcome and/or the potential benefits or disadvantages for one's own or others' physical, emotional or financial well-being.

Risky behaviors can occur in different settings. As a person grows old and he is exposed to different situations, his access to perilous situations changes. For example, a person who is aware of the consequences of excessive alcohol consumption will eventually detach himself from this habit. This either can be because he himself has experienced the cost of this behavior or he has seen some around him suffering because of it.

However, this is different when it comes to adolescents and teenagers. Since they are in their growing age and have not been exposed much to the outside world, they have an urge to get involved in certain behaviors that may lead to unfavorable outcomes. Teenagers can engage in a variety of dangerous activities, but because the use of technology has increased dramatically over the past 20 years, taking risks in an online setting is a relatively new thing.

It has been seen that the emotional and psychological well-being of children has been affected in a dangerous way since risk-taking in an online setting has become common. There are many instances were teenagers have involved themselves in activities like cyberbullying and hacking that has eventually caused great harm to the victims of it. These victims eventually involve themselves in self-harm, while the predator spends the rest of his life dodging the punishment.

If dig deeper into this topic we will find many different types of research that touch upon the different areas related to risk behavior. Below I have explained some of the published research on the topic:

Research # 1

The first research that we will be discussing in this chapter is regarding Risk behavior in adolescents and it focuses on the area of drug use and sexual activity, which was proposed by Silvia Ciairano. It is a cross-national study that compares the risk behaviors of adolescents belonging to Italy and the Netherlands.

The major aim of this study was to compare the Italian and Dutch samples of adolescents in order to determine the differences and the similarities in them when it comes to risky behavior. However, to conduct this research an extensive questionnaire was prepared and was given out to the young adults of Italy and the Netherlands. From this questionnaire, the measures of risk behaviors, related attitudes, cognitions and models, and protective and risk factors were inferred.

The results of this research showed that despite there are differences in the cultural scripts, social policies and laws about sex and drug use in both countries still their involvement in drugs and sexual activity is still the same. This means that the culture of the policies of a country has nothing to do with the risky behaviors of young adults. It is their psychological and emotional urge to do something that they are generally stopped from.

Research #2

Another research on this topic covers the area of risk behaviorand health Knowledge. It was conducted by PA Cook and MA Bellis and both of them belonged to the Public Health sector ofLiverpool, UK.

The major aim behind this research was to identify whether there is a relationship between risk behavior and the knowledge of health among the public. So, in order to investigate this, a questionnaire was distributed which was filled by 472 anonymous students. However, for this study Risk-taking behavior was measured as the number of different risk behaviors undertaken in the previous 12 months. While knowledge and perception were said to be measured by the degree to which subjects agreed with statements of risk-related information. These ranged in complexity from straightforward assertions that connected a particular activity with a health risk to precise declarations that quantified the strength of such correlations.

As a result of this study, it was found that risk-taking behavior was the most among those who belonged to younger age groups, were males, had parents in non-manual occupations, and believed in God. Overall, no significant relationship between Knowledge and risk-taking behavior was found. However, risk-taking was positively related to more accurate responses to numerical risk questions and risk-takers were also more likely to perceive both voluntary and involuntary risks as less risky.

Research #3

Another research belonging to the area of risk behavior that we will be discussing in this chapter is "High-risk behavior in hypomanic states". This study was proposed by Kathryn Fletcher, Gordon Parker, Amelia Paterson, and Howe Synnott, in the year 2012. However, it has been identified in research from the past that people get involved in risk-taking activities when they are in a hypomanic state, but before this study, there was no such discussion on the potential harm that comes with these activities. The study that we will be discussing in this chapter examines risk-taking behaviors and their consequences in those individuals who have a bipolar II condition.

In order to conduct this research Participants were called from Black Dog Institute Depression Clinic, that is based in Sydney. These participants were then asked to complete a series of questions that were related to their previous risk-taking behaviors during their hypomanic states. A total of 98 samples were collected and then analyzed.

The results of this study showed that during hypomanic states people involved themselves in risky activities like excessive drug or alcohol use, endangering sexual activities, dangerous driving, and overspending. Key consequences included financial burden, interpersonal conflict, and feelings of shame, remorse, and guilt. Less than one-fifth of participants felt that hypomania should be treated due to the hazards involved, despite the fact that they were aware of the risks and negative effects connected with hypomanic behaviors.

Types of Risk Behavior and Their Leading Consequences

There are many different types of risk behaviors that can be seen among both the teenagers as well as grownup adults. I have explained a few of them along with the consequences of each.

• Behaviors leading to Unintentional Injuriesand Violence

There are certain risk behaviors that might lead an individualto unintentional injuries. The best example of this type of risky behavior is, using a cell phone while driving. Though it has been strictly prohibited in the traffic laws of all the countries around the world, still is a very common practice. People use their cell phones while driving and then they end up facing an accident that causes unintentional injuries to them. Other behaviors of such kind include riding in cars with drivers that are drunk, riding a bike without a helmet, and not wearing a seat belt when riding as a passenger in a car.

Apart from this, if I talk about behaviors among teens that lead to violence, then they could be, being in a physical fight, being physically hurt by a girlfriend or boyfriend, experiencing bullying, experiencing being hit, carrying a weapon, avoiding school because of its lack of safety and lastly, considering and/or attempting suicide.

• **Sexual Behaviors Leading to Sexually transmitted Diseases and Unwanted Pregnancies**

Another type of risk behavior is being involved in unprotected sexual activities this can include, having multiple partners, having unprotected sex, having sex before the age of 13, not being tested for STDs, and also, consuming alcohol or drugs before or during the intercourse. All these behaviors ultimately lead to unfavorable situations like unwanted pregnancies and even getting sexually transmitted diseases.

This behavior is quite common among young adults as they don't think before diving into anything. They believe that getting involved in such activities will give them pleasure and will also make them feel good about themselves, but they completely ignore the cost of it. However, adults on the other hand try to protect themselves from such behaviors as they are aware of the consequences.

- **Drug and alcohol abuse leading to addiction**

Another risky behavior that we generally see is alcohol and drug abuse. Usually, people consume alcohol or drugs as a one- time thing, but then eventually it becomes a very important part of their life. It affects their productivity levels, their relationships, and lastly their own wellbeing. But, unfortunately, by then it is very late for them to detach themselves from it and turn towards a happy and healthy life.

- **Vaping & Tobacco Use leading to Health Issues**

The fourth type of risk behavior is smoking tobacco and vaping. Behaviors that lead to tobacco use include smoking a complete cigarette before turning 13, vaping, experimenting with cigarette smoking, smoking a cigarette at least once a week, and using various forms of smokeless tobacco. Nowadays vaping has become a significant problem among teens as they believe that it is not as harmful as an actual cigarette but unfortunately it is not right. Research have proven that vaping can have a medium to drastic impact on the physical as well as mental health of those who engage themselves in this practice.

- **Unhealthy Dietary Behaviors**

Although we don't consider unhealthy dietary habits as risky behavior they are. When we don't take care of our health, we are exposing our bodies to thousands of health risks and are causing serious harm to our wellbeing. However, it has been seen that in the past few years such behavior has increased and people have ultimately stopped paying attention to their health. They have involved themselves in unhealthy dietary behaviors, by giving a reason that they have no time to take care of their health, in thisfast-paced world.

If we talk about risky behaviors when it comes to unhealthy dietary habits then it can include, skipping breakfast, not consuming an adequate amount of vegetables and fruits, drinking sugary drinks and sodas, not drinking milk, and not drinking enough amounts of fresh fruit juices.

- ## Inadequate Physical Activity

Lack of physical activity is risky behavior that can result in poor physical health. Risk factors for this include not engaging in any cardio activity in the previous week, skipping physical education classes, spending three hours or more a day playing video games or on the computer, and binge-watching television.

Although it is normal for adolescents to explore, it can be dangerous when some of these teens' risky behavior becomes routine. In relation to the risky behaviors mentioned above, the CDC keeps track of the leading causes of death among teenagers. For instance, in 2010, there were 4,678 homicides,

4,600 suicides, and 12,341 unintentional injury deaths amongadolescents between the ages of 15 and 24.

Impact of Risky behavior on Emotionalwellbeing

Physically risky behaviors like skydiving can impress people and provide opportunities for lively conversations and a connection with more adventurous people, but unhealthy, violent, illegal, or risky behaviors can alienate people. They can make a person detach himself from the outside world because the repercussions of his risky behavior don't allow him to face the world. This can make his emotional and psychological health worse to such an extent that he might need to seek professional help.

If we talk about risky behavior, then its impact on emotionalhealth is the more neglected area. There isn't any sufficient discussion on how these risky behaviors can actually jeopardize the emotional well-being of a person. However, in this section,I will be discussing different risky behaviors and how they can negatively impact a person's emotional well-being.

- ### **Getting involved in online Crimes**

Over the past few years, it has been seen that online crimes have increased. Youngsters who have access to technology and are knowledgeable about the different I.T. systems usually take undue advantage. They commit online crimes because they know they won't be caught that easily. By online crimes, I mean hacking, cyberbullying, and blackmailing someone with their private information.

But, one thing they don't consider is that with time they also suffer because of their risky actions. They constantly fear that they might get caught for what they have done or even remain in prison for the rest of their lives. This ultimately takes a great toll on their emotional well-being, making them mentally and psychologically sick.

- ### **Gaining weight**

Even though generally people don't consider gaining weight a risky behavior, but it is. When we are in our younger years of life, we eat without paying attention to our weight. That is the time when we consume junk or unhealthy foods and pay little to no attention to our physical activity. But, once we grow out of that age and our body starts showing the effects of our unhealthy eating, we become depressed. We no longer like ourselves, and our self-esteem drops to the level of zero. That is the moment when our emotional well-being gets affected to quite a serious level.

Emotional and Psychological Wellbeing

This brings me to the point that emotional being stems from our psychological well-being. If a person is doing fine psychologically and has no mental health issues, only then would he be able to keep his emotional well-being in check. This means that if a person is not depressed or facing any mental health issue, only then he will be able to control his feelings, thoughts, and behaviors.

Here I would share an example of two sisters, Anna and Amelia who were grown in the same household, but their psychological was different. Anna would always be ready to take risks. She liked going out with friends and living her life the most. But the only thing she lacked was control over her actions and thoughts. She could be easily lured into activities that could be extremely risky for her.

However, Amelia on the other hand was mentally and emotionally sound. She knew what to do and what not to do.

Shewas aware of her actions and the repercussions that they would lead to. Therefore, this was the reason why she never got involved in any risky activity.

This brings me to the point that it is purely our psychologicaland emotional state that makes us attracted to risky behavior. Ifsomeone knows how to control his or her emotions and is able to express their feelings in an appropriate way then there are very less chances of them doing something that is uncertain.

Also, your ability to work efficiently and handle life's difficulties depends on your emotional well-being. You might be able to reach your maximum potential. It enables you to collaborate with others and give back to the community.

Your physical health is also impacted. According to research, a positive outlook on life is associated with outward manifestations of health. These include a healthier weight, lower blood pressure, and a lower risk of heart disease.

CHAPTER 12

IMPROVING EMOTIONAL WELL-BEING

The world that we live in today, requires us to perform multiple functions at the same time. Our everyday routines are so packed that we don't even a few minutes to reflect upon our physical mental or emotional health. However, this is the reasonwhy today we hear so many young people losing their lives because of health issues like cardiac arrests and depression.

It is high time that we work towards the elimination of the things that take a toll on our metal and emotional health and leave at the verge of losing our lives. So, in this chapter, I will be discussing different ways through which an individual can not only improve his mental wellbeing but also maintain it for longer period of time. Although it requires quite a lot of time andeffort but in the end, it is all totally worth it.

Ways to improve emotional well being

As humans, we experience tens of emotions in a day. Some people easily get carried away by these emotions, while some know how to manage them and stay focused in their lives.

However, the people who can easily manage their thoughts, emotions, and actions have better emotional resilience and lead peaceful life. Below I have explained a few ways through which you can take control of your feeling and emotions and also stay resilient.

- **Move your body**

The first way through which you can take control of your emotions is that you move your body after every 90 minutes.In this way, your mind will remain distracted from the thoughts that trouble you, and you can get involved in something productive. By moving your body, I don't mean that you need to do some hardcore exercise after every 90 minutes. You can just walk around the house, dance to your favorite music, put away the laundry, or just go outside for a brisk walk.

In this way, you will feel active and will also feel that you have done something productive for yourself and your physical, mental, and emotional health.

- **Have a proper routine**

Having a proper routine will help you do everything on time. In this way, you will be able to balance everything that you want to do in life with your work. You can include some time for your self-care, some time for your hobbies, and some time for your family. Through this, you will not regret missing out on anything in life, and your emotional well-being will alsoremain in check.

However, those who constantly struggle to manage everything together and have no proper routine eventually make their mental and emotional health suffer. Apart from this, they always stay unhappy in life because they can't pursue their hobbies, they don't have time to take care of themselves, and they have also ignored their family.

- **Connect with people around you**

Another way through which you can improve your emotional well-being is by connecting with people around you. When you talk to people who have a positive mindset, or we can say a growth mindset, we automatically start feeling better, we get to learn a lot from them, and we try to implementthe same changes in our life as well. So, in order to be emotionally healthy, we should spend time with people who bring quality to our life. We must be closer to the people who make us feel good about ourselves and also give us the confidence to step out of our comfort zones.

Similarly, if you make yourself available to those who need your help and who want to share their problems with you, then you must do that. This is yet another way through which you will feel accomplished, and your emotional health will also flourish.

• **Learn to Forgive**

Holding grudges against people can only make your mental and emotional, and emotional health worse Forgive. Therefore, if you really want to be an emotionally healthy person, then you should learn to forgive people. No matterhow big their mistake is or how much they have hurt you, you should always let it go and move forward in life. Forgiveness frees you to keep your power, and it opens the path to live in the moment. So, always choose the option of forgiveness allows for happiness and growth.

- ## Get involved in Welfare work

Doing something for others has always been the best way to feel at peace. So, those who are striving hard to give a boost to their emotional health should consider doing something for society. This can be something as little as planting a tree or as big as providing a needy person financial help. But the condition is that this act must be truly selfless. You should not expect to be repaid for your good deed or be appreciated by the society as this is the only way through which you will feel happy. Some of the common welfare acts can be, picking up groceries for your neighbor. Volunteering at school that teaches children with special abilities or being kind to people around.

- ## Get a sound sleep

To achieve the goal of emotional wellbeing, you must pay attention to your sleep schedule. Having a sound sleep of eight hours can help your body to repair itself. Also, it refreshes the brain to manage memories and process information. Therefore, it can be said that those who get a sound sleep everyday are more likely to have better emotional and mental health.

Additionally, having a proper sleep schedule is also very important. By this I mean that you should get to bed at the same time every day and similarly wake up at the same time too. This will bring uniformity and focus in your life. Also, you wake up in a better mood with makes you spend your daysin a lot better way.

- **Be kind to yourself**

Among all the ways to improve emotional wellbeing, treating yourself right is the most important one. If you pay attention to yourself and be kind to yourself then it will give you enough confidence to take care of your emotions and your thoughts. So, ask yourself what gives you joy? What space youfeel happy being in? And most importantly, what brings peace to you? Once you answer these questions and implement it in your life, a lot of your issues will be solved and you will leada happier and peaceful life.

- **Be self-aware**

Lastly, being aware of your actions, thoughts habits and character traits makes you emotionally well. When you know what you like and what you don't like then it will be easier for you to choose the best options and this will bring you emotional peace. For example, are person who has identified it over the years that he does not like being around the people who are toxic and talk about themselves only, then you willtry to distant yourself from them. You will avoid going to the gathering where such people are invited and also you willblock them on your social media handles. In this way to will stay away from those people and will be in an emotionally healthy space.

Once you improve your emotional wellbeing, the urge of getting involved in risky behaviors will also be eliminated. As you will get control of your emotions and your feelings it will get much easier for you to detach yourself from the thoughts of doing something that can bring unfavorable consequences.

Better Physical and Mental Health Impacts Emotional Well-Being Positively

Mental and physical health are intricately linked. Both physical and mental health problems can result from injuries. In addition to boosting mood and reducing stress, physical activity and a good diet also have positive effects on mental health. Long-term psychological benefits of physical health are felt by the individual. Physical activity improves mental wellness, according to the American

Heart Association. Regular exercise can help to reduce stress, anxiety, despair, and anger.

Our emotional, psychological, and social well-being are all parts of our mental health. It influences our thoughts, emotions, and behaviors. Additionally, it influences how we respond to stress, interact with others, and make decisions. Every period of life, from childhood and adolescence to maturity, is vital for mental health.

If you have mental health issues, they may have an impact on your thinking, mood, and behavior over the course of your life. Therefore, it can be said that if a person has better mental and physical health then his emotional wellbeing will also be impacted positively. He would feel better about himself and would face little to zero problems in his life.

Emotional stability in life through multiple Activities

Though it is difficult to achieve emotional wellbeing in life but it is even more difficult to maintain it over a longer period of time. Usually people get off track and stop working towards their emotional health, and this eventually brings them to the same stage from where they initially started. However, in section of the chapter I will be discussing a few activities that can help you maintain your emotional health for a longer period of time and will also bring stability in your action.

- **Check on yourself Multiple times**

When you are working towards the goal of maintain your emotional wellbeing, you should check on yourself multiple times. It can be explained in such a way that a portion of your response to whatever stimulus is in front of you is unconscious. When you step on a LEGO, your foot hurts and you get upset at the same time. Similarly, you become nervous as you watch the outrageous news. This means that before your logical mind has a chance to keep up, those thoughts and feelings will come to you. Therefore, take a moment to check in with yourself and determine what you are focusing on at least twice or three times a day. See what the emotions are bringing up by keeping that attention. Are you anxious because you're concentrating on the unpleasant events occurring, or are you ecstatic about the prospects that lie ahead?

Most individuals are unaware of the fact that, out of a subconscious desire to survive, our minds are always focused on all the bad things happening. These unfavorable emotions might easily overpower everything else when you're operating on autopilot. However, by consciously becoming aware of your thoughts and feelings, you can choose to deliberately change your attention and break the habit of operating automatically. You may give yourself the information you need to understand why you feel the way you do and where your attention is during the day by checking in with yourself several times a day.

- **Don't Make Your Emotions "Wrong"**

Your emotions serve as a feedback mechanism for how you perceive your current environment. You think that your current condition shouldn't be happening to you if you prove them wrong. At that point, you start contesting reality and searching for someone or something to blame. We have this misconception that we shouldn't feel a certain way or that recognizing our feelings makes us weak. By accepting that you are not your thoughts, feelings, or emotions, you open yourself up to hearing criticism and learning from it rather than reacting to it.

- **Acknowledge your thoughts and emotions**

Your ability to identify the trigger behind a thought or

feeling depends on your ability to recognize your emotions and thoughts. As I previously stated, our subconscious mind is continuously preoccupied with unfavorable feelings and thoughts, especially in the morning. If you don't acknowledge those emotions, the rest of the day will be spent struggling. Because your brain acts as though you're fighting an opponent and your body uses energy fighting itself, your brain will release the stress hormone cortisol.

According to studies, simply noticing negative thoughts and understanding that it's natural for your brain to be in a reactionary mode offers you the power to decide to change your perspective and pay attention to the opportunity rather than the issue. Instead than attempting to correct them, be more conscious of them. It's not necessary for you to "correct" your feelings. Not the feeling itself, but the thing that caused you to feel that way, needs to be fixed.

- **Win the battle in your mind before it becomesreal**

The majority of our worries and tensions are brought on by what we imagine might occur. The terror often simply exists in our minds and is not genuine. The worst-case scenarios are all imagined in the future and are motivated by some form of past suffering. Our assurance is undermined by the sense of being trapped between an unchangeable past and an uncertain future. All the other feelings are amplified by that feeling of helplessness. However, the secret weapon is that, by using your intellect, you can also triumph in those conflicts.

- **Feel your emotions fully**

Lastly, feel your emotions fully. Humans continuously criticize themselves and don't allow themselves to experience their feelings fully. Like the relief that occasionally mingles with despair. Because we believe we shouldn't feel a certain way, our emotions can drive us to feel guilty and ashamed. The shame and guilt keep us from developing our potential. The triggers are present because the emotions are present, and you cannot just interrupt that circuit. Instead, you must finish the circuit and experience all of the feelings.

When we allow ourselves to experience the emotion, that's when we're shedding light on the situation. Our energy-suckingworry and uncertainty will start to lose strength.

Emotional Stability in Life through Exercise

Apart from adding some activities in your everyday life, you must add some physical exercises that can help you maintain your emotional wellbeing. These exercises are explained below

- **Mediation**

While you can practice mindfulness at any moment, meditation is a more regimented activity. Since there are usually no outside distractions, you can concentrate on a single subject, such as your breath, an object in particular, or a mantra. You may find it more effective to control your overall stress if you schedule frequent meditation sessions during specified times. Research on meditation suggests that the practice may carry a number of benefits, like better overall mood, less depression and anxiety and reduced insomnia.

It is said that practicing mediation on everyday basis can increase the feelings of self- kindness and self-acceptance, while also reducing the thoughts regarding self-criticism

Because mindfulness meditation is structured, you

must set out a specific period of time to settle in and pay attention. Mindfulness meditation generally encourages you to focus on your body and breathe while observing your thoughts as they come and go.

- **Exercise**

It goes without saying that keeping your body active will make you feel better both physically and mentally. Exercise is a terrific strategy to maintain a more stable emotional system in addition to fighting a variety of physical health issues linked to BPD. 7 If you don't already have an exercise regimen, think about talking to your doctor first to find out which kind of exercise are most suitable for you. After that, you can start your personal fitness regimen by following these steps:

- Don't start big; start modest. If you are eager to begin, you can push yourself too far and put yourself in danger of getting hurt. Instead, experiment with gradually lengthening and/or toughening your workouts over time.

- Experiment with different types of exercise. You can find the exercise form that you prefer by trying out a range of activities; this will increase your likelihood of sticking with it. You can discover that you enjoy working out alone more than with a team, or that you find entertainment in group activities.

•   Incorporate relaxation exercises into your routine. Consider including relaxing exercises like yoga or tai chi into your workout routine in addition to strength training and cardio. These exercises integrate controlled breathing with activity, and they could be useful for reducing stress.

CHAPTER 13

AN INTRODUCTION TO SOCIAL WELL-BEING

Humans are social beings. They cannot survive all alone. It isan instinct that individuals engage and connect, forming a mutual bond. This is what gives them a sense of belongingness to each other. However, social connections can never be forced. They typically develop with time and process without much effort.

Think of a best friend in your workspace. Did you go to him and asked to be your friend immediately? No, it happens with time. Did you have no one else except him in your workplace? No, we have so many other individuals working side by side butnot each becomes a friend. It is because, with certain people, you feel more connected. You like them, spend more time and share your personal stuff. It makes you both connect to a deeper level. They are the ones you trust and prefer to get into a relationship with. On the other hand, other people also exist. You might know them but don't have a deeper connection to them. Both sorts of relationships significantly affect a person's social well- being.

Social well-being refers to creating and developing healthyinterpersonal relations among individuals.

Social well-being is an individual's status regarding his connections. It includes both the human interaction as well as the surrounding effects. The phenomenon of social well-being ismore focused on not only developing yet sustaining social relationships. A meaningful relationship can bring positivity and happiness. Hence, it aims to make an individual feel valued while consistently feeling part of or cared for.

Salient Aspects of Social Well-being

Social well-being revolves around a healthy picture of human relationships. However, it relies on multiple pointers, which work all together to make it a success. Some of the essential aspects of social well-being may include the following,

• Maintaining two-way communication that iscomfortable and easy-going.

• Developing a meaningful, healthy relationshipthat is beneficial for both.

• Connecting while respecting personal

boundariesof each other.

-                               Treating with kindness and gratitude.

Social well-being is a significant element of an individual's overall health. How can a person stay content while he has a broken relationship? No matter how physically and mentally fit a person is, even a slight disturbance in his social connections can affect his social and overall well-being.

Having the ability to keep up with their social connections boosts your emotional well-being. It makes you feel supported. It additionally encourages you to live a happier life.

Factors Affecting Social Well-being

According to the World Health Organization (WHO), social well-being is an essential dimension of health besides physical and mental aspects. It plays a critical role in improving the quality of life. It ensures your social performance and efficacy.

Keeping up with social well-being is very critical in every phase of life. Imagine you are bad at making connections or carrying your relationships for the long term. It will affect not only your social existence but also your body's health and life. Being unable to keep up with social relations causes loneliness. When a person becomes alone, it further leads to depression and other psychological conditions. It can eventually result in healthdeterioration.

Maintaining social well-being is crucial. However, it becomes pretty challenging at times. Several factors affect the social well-being of an individual. Some of them are described below;

- **Low Self Esteem**

The primary factor of poor social well-being can be an individual's low self-esteem. It stimulates a person to doubt himself and the relationship. People with low confidence when they get into a relationship fail to persist with it. They either lookdown upon themselves or cannot tolerate others' goodness. Therefore, it results in causing various conflicts, weakening therelationship.

Focus on building up your self-confidence. You are who youare. No one can take away what is meant for you. Believe in yourcapabilities and never hesitate to take risks.

- **Lack of Time**

In today's rapidly paced world, everyone is busy doing this orthat. It isn't easy to make time for even vital things. Social well- being turns out to be positive and extraordinary only when given time. Therefore, reduced time can be an important factor in influencing social well-being.

People lack time-managing skills. Even though they have spare time, they do not know how to make the most of it. Unlikethem, you must make time for your family, friends, and relationships.

- **Poor Understanding**

A relationship, whether it's between a mother-daughter, friend-friend, or anyone, is always a two-sided thing. You cannot expect someone to be understanding while becoming intolerant of it. There is a need to understand the reasons and give some personal space. The bonding that lacks theunderstanding required can also affect social well-being.

Importance of Social Well-being

Maintaining optimal social well-being is significant for

multiple reasons. Having stable relationships with your family, friends, and colleagues lets you work productively. You feel comfortable with who you are. It encourages you to interact with people more positively. The support you have from your social relations boosts your self-esteem. Whatever the difficulty comes in, you have someone there to back you. This motivation makes you overcome the challenges and move ahead in life, achieving your dream goals.

Good social well-being enables you to think and act clearly. It lets you create boundaries among the connected and other individuals. You can identify the available ones and set limits to avoid falling into conflicts.

Why does Social Well-being matter?

Social well-being also plays a crucial part in improving your emotional capability. It keeps you healthy physically, mentally, and emotionally. If a person is dealing with a broken friendship or relationship trauma, it will definitely make him sad and depressed. Even though the bond breakage has no direct contact with his physical health, the declining social well-being can cause mental or even physical ailments. For example, you must have heard of someone who attempted suicide just because of a relationship breakup.

Stress and physical harm are common among teenagers. It is because their social well-being is not strong enough to keep up with relationships positively. They have more chances of fluctuation. Youngsters can easily make or break a connection or relationship. Despite seeming very easy or ineffective, it can cause unimaginable impacts on their lives.

Emphasis on sustaining social well-being increased in recent years. The lack of social contact can adversely affect an individual's health. Do you ever sit alone and randomly start
criticizing yourself? Sometimes, in loneliness, our brain highlights our negative points. It changes our perspectives about ourselves and triggers us to hate.

Research has even proved that being alone is terrible. If a person sits alone for a long time, it induces a person toward negative activities. However, living in complete isolation brings out negative health consequences.

Benefits of Social Well-being

Social well-being is always worthy. Building and maintaining positive relationships proffers you the subsequent advantages;

- **Behavioral**

Social bonding with friends, family, and colleagues affects our behavior. It tends to engage us more in positive talk rather than drowning away with negative emotions. The positive behavior makes us intriguing to other people, leading to further connections. It also improves our body health.

- **Psychosocial**

Keeping up with our social well-being encourages us to stay strong mentally. It distances us from stressing factors and prevents emotional turmoil. Hence, social well-being boosts our psychological capability. It positively influences our mental health.

- **Physiological**

Social well-being lets individuals stay relaxed and content. When a person is satisfied with relations, it makes him feel better. Engaging and connecting to love ones positively promotes health. As a result of which, our life's longevity increases.

Positive social well-being upgrades the lifestyle. It offers a more positive outlook, changing the lifestyle to a healthier one.

Measuring Elements of Social Well-being According to research, social well-being is composed of two main elements.

- **Social Adjustment** - It is a combination of satisfaction in relationships, performance in social roles, and adjustment to the environment.

- **Social Support** - The number of people in contact and their satisfaction.

Consequently, an individual can determine his social well-being using the two ways. If you are good with the relationships and people you have, you are sound. You can also check if you have difficulty fulfilling your social responsibilities or adapting to your surroundings. If yes, you might have an adjustment problem in maintaining social well-being.

How many people support you at the moment? Ask yourself. There can be 2,3,4,5, or more. Are you satisfied with that many people, or do you need more? The answer can let you know if your social well-being needs to improve or is already stable.

How to Improve Your Social Well-being?
Since social well-being is crucial to work upon, you must be wondering how to. There can be multiple ways to improve your social health. Nonetheless, the primary step is to be aware of yourself. You must realize the significance of social well-being. When you fully agree with the idea and know its worth for your overall health, you will find it easy to enhance your social well-being.

Taking specific measures for physical and mental health is expected. Likewise, you can make specific changes, add positives, and neglect negatives for social well-being. It might seem odd to you because of its unpopularity, but the efforts will be worth it.

- ## Engage & Connect

Social beings (humans) are the asset of social well-being. Almost every individual hesitates to talk at first. But those who take the initiative are the confident ones. You will find yourself in a new place, among unique faces at numerous phases of life. Rather than fearing to interact, you should feel free to adapt. Whether a new school, college, workspace, or whatever, there is a need to communicate and engage. It is not necessary to be with everyone, but there always can be few to connect with.

Be confident, take the initiative, and create social connections. They can only lead to strong social relations, which can sometimes be helpful.

- ## Prioritize Your Well-being

While maintaining social well-being, one of the risks is losing your health by other means. Excess to anything is bad. Likewise, the extra efforts of forcing healthy relationships and support can turn out to you. When you push yourself so much to focus on others, there is a chance you neglect yourself.

Remember, even in an emergency; the instructions are to

wear your oxygen mask first before helping anyone else. You should also prioritize your health and well-being before doing anything extra for someone. No doubt, helping others overcome trauma or trouble is good. But while doing so, try not to make yourself end up on a similar note.

- **Stay Active with Friends & Family**

Making connections is super easy; however, keeping up with them is challenging. You can connect to many people in your college or university, but you will hardly find yourself talking to or caring about each of them. That is why having a smaller yet valuable social circle is always preferable. Even with that, try to stay active and spend quality time with your family and friends. It is vital for your social well-being. The more you engage, and open up about things, the deeper your relationship becomes.

Every time something good or bad happens, we want to tell it first to our loved ones. Talking and staying connected to them proves to be therapy for us. This practice either directly or indirectly enhances our social well-being multiple times.

- ## **Volunteer for Community**

Volunteering is a healthy activity. It engages you in something positive while building an impact. Giving yourself an opportunity to work for the sake of societal benefits enriches a sense of social responsibility in you.

Doing a job is a must; however, volunteering is a choice. It drives positive energy. Working together with other individuals also provides you with a chance to exchange thoughts.

CHAPTER 14

SOCIAL DEVELOPMENT & THE
INDIVIDUAL JOURNEY

Individuals are a significant element of society. The relationship among individuals such as family members, friends, neighbors, or work colleagues constitutes a meaningful society. Without human relationships, a society is nothing but a materialistic structure. It cannot develop or succeed at all.

The progress of a society is always linked to its individuals' well-being. If a person is physically, mentally, or emotionally weak, he cannot work efficiently. It will eventually affect society. Likewise, if an individual lacks the basic ethics of behaving and interacting within a community, it affects progressand the societal environment.

Social development is defined as individual well-being to reach their potential for the benefit of society.

Social development is a process of individual learning involving positive behavioral and attitude changes over time. As an individual grows, he can better understand his individuality within the community. He learns how to interact and communicate with other people. It also encourages him to liveand adapt to his surroundings.

Social development is more about how a person develops hisinterpersonal relations at a community level. It includes relationships with family, neighbors, friends, colleagues, and others. The way an individual responds to conflicts shows his development level.

Social Development in Children

Social development is a crucial yet never-ending process. It begins in a person's early childhood and continues as a life-long learning process. A child, when born, knows nothing about his surroundings or the world. He has no idea how to behave and function within a society. However, he learns the basics from his home, family, and siblings. It shapes a child's behavior, attitude,and perceptions.

For example, a child watches his siblings fighting with each other. One of his parents comes, dissolves the quarrel, and advises the children never to fight again. From this scenario, a child must have learned that fighting is bad and that he shouldn'tdo this.

This is one example, and there can be many more. Reflect on your childhood; who has taught you greeting? How many times save elders asked you to behave well? Speak nicely or do this or that. Each of these things that we as individuals learn from others and society is a part of the process. They help us grow and mature while being socially responsible human beings.

Research & Studies Indicating Social Development in Children

Social development states that children experience life, observe the actions and responses of others, and from them, theylearn how to act or behave within society.

Our earliest experiences stick to us for years or even for life. They even influence our adult decisions. It means whatever we learn or go through as children will remain there. This is what signifies the importance of social development in a child.

Since a child is incapable, the early years' social developmentresponsibility falls onto the parents' shoulders. They play a vital role in shaping a child's personality. In fact, how parents behave in one's childhood affects his life for decades.

According to a study in Child Development, the researchers found that the emotional support a child receives during the early 3 ½ years of his life has an effect on his education, social life, and romantic relationships for 20 or 30 years later. It claims that children raised in supportive and caring home environments tend to do better as adults. They perform well in schools and attain higher education degrees. They are more likely to get along with their peers and relationships.

A parent-child relationship is very critical, especially in the early years. Parents need to communicate positively with a child as much as they can. They are supposed to be there in a child's success or failure. No matter what, parents should be the cheerleaders. These little interactions are vital for a child's healthy social development. However, parental behavior is only one factor influencing that. It may not necessarily give visible outcomes, but it thoroughly benefits the process.

As per another Child Developmental study, children's early life experiences can let others predict if they can develop a social anxiety disorder. The parent's separation is the major reason for such stress and instability. The children who live

The study results show that sensitive children who face such incidents feel more anxious while socializing. They typically avoid gatherings and parties. All these behaviors are genuine and understandable. They can affect social development negatively. However, it can be treated through psychological and behavioraltherapies.

Why Is Social Development SoImportant?

Social development has been vital since childhood. It can impact an individual's life in many ways. If a person lacks the ability to interact with people, it seizes his growth opportunities. For example, children who are underdeveloped socially remain submissive. They are usually shy or unconfident to speak on their behalves. When they lack decision-making power, they are more likely to be affected by peer pressure.

Every individual begins developing socially from an early age. Whatever a child learns or adapts stays there for a lifetime. That is why focusing on your child's social development is necessary.

Helping a child to develop stronger socially can be essential for subsequent reasons;

- ## To Boost Self-Esteem

Letting a child play and engage with other children is very important. It enables him to experience and explores different situations. It encourages him to be confident while reinforcing his individuality. Children who are more social and playful become more interactive adults. They have healthier friend circles that ensure a high self-esteem level.

- ## To Strengthen Learning Skills

Having a healthy relationship with peers helps children adjust easily. It strengthens their ability to understand and adapt to different situations. Those children who have a hard time getting on with their classmates at an early age are expected to face similar difficulties in their adult life. It affects their communication skills, declining their socializing ability.

- ## To Improve Language

Children with more interaction opportunities excel. While playing, when they engage with their age-fellows or even elders, their communication ability enhances. Consistent talk improves their grip over the language. It brings more positive socialdevelopment. A child who knows how to ask or say what he wants is intelligent. He, as an adult, can better react and respondthan others.

- ### To Promote Positive Attitude

A nurtured and cared for child develops into a positive social being. He is well aware of the values, culture, and behaviors. It enables him to cater to his relationships in a positive way. Hence, it eventually brings peace and happiness to his life.

Factors Affecting Social Development

Social development is based on multiple phases of an individual's life and, therefore, involves numerous factors. Some of the most prominent factors affecting the process are following;

- ### Home & Family

Family is considered the first socializing agency. It is from where almost every individual begins life. That is why the home environment and family largely affect the process of social development. The child imitates the behavior of his parents or other family members. Thus, he consciously or unconsciously builds good or bad habits.

If a child's upbringing takes place in a happy, more positive family culture, he becomes socially active and healthy. On the other hand, if a child grows up in a negative environment where he has not been looked after carefully by the family, he must remain behind. The trauma a child faces in childhood remains there forever. It limits his growing ability. Therefore, ensuring a safe and sound home environment for a child's healthy growth is essential.

- ## Cultural & Society

The society and culture in which an individual lives play a vital role. Societal culture influences a person's values, actions, behavior, thinking, and almost every characteristic. Hence, individuals coming from different societies and cultures reflect other behaviors. The level of one's social development relies upon his surrounding culture. A person who belongs to a privileged community will be more informed than anyone else.

- ## Socio-Economic Status

The class/status of a family matters a lot. A child developed in a low-class or low-income family differs greatly from one grown in a high-status rich family. According to research results, 10% of a child's academic achievement correlates with the quality of their home life at the age of three.

Children with rich parents can afford high schools, rich friend circles, lavish gatherings, and everything superior. The expensive schools and luxuries make them grow socially stronger compared to other children. His socializing skills improve naturally when a youngster meets and engages with different individuals. He adapts his communication style, language, and other skills. Thus, such children develop strongersocially as well as emotionally.

- ### Love & Affection

A child, when born, is a tender little human being. He more or less remains fragile. In the early years, love and affection are the necessities of a child. If treated lovingly, a child feels more secure. It enables him to develop socially and emotionally. When supported by the family, a kid easily gives in to relationships outside. He makes friends and associates, expecting to give and take a similar level of love and affection. It altogether contributes to an individual's social development inan ideal way.

- **School Programs**

Educational Institutions are potent agencies of social development. In school, individual gets a chance to mingle and grow with a diversified group of students. He takes part in activities promoting social communication. Teachers in schools encourage individuals to develop healthy habits. Each of the little to huge things in school impacts social development.

- **Peer Group**

A peer group satisfies several individual needs. Whether it be acceptance, rejection, fame, affection, belongingness, etc., aperson can expect it all from his peers. If someone becomes lucky enough to have a good peer group at an early age, he can possibly adopt good behavior and characteristics.

- **Social Participation**

As a child grows and becomes a youngster, he realizes his social responsibility. Taking part in social activities has always been helpful for individuals. It helps individuals widen their social circle, making new contacts and relationships. It additionally adds to their social understanding. While working in different social settings, a person learns a lot. It gives him an opportunity to develop various skills such as leadership, cooperation, and tolerance.

Participating socially also brings self-consciousness. It multiplies the level of social development an individual has.

3 Aspects of Social Development

There are three different aspects of social development.

- **Social Aspects**

Today, almost every society is getting more modern day by day. Traditional societal culture does not exist anymore. Everything is getting more digitalized. Likewise, individuals are socializing more on virtual platforms rather than physical ones. It is all because individuals are getting more socially developed than ever before. Unlike earlier, communities are working more democratically than authoritatively. People now have a right to vote or even raise their voices. They have the power to choose their leaders. They are more socially aware.

Social status does not come along with a child by birth.

Each individual has to achieve it through hard work, effort, and positive behavior. That is only possible due to social development. Another important benefit of social development enhancing social aspects is the changing structure of families. Nowadays, people prefer nuclear families. Due to such small family systems, child development gets easier. The children have stronger bonding and sustainable relationships.

- **Cultural Aspects**

With social development, people's attitudes within a society have become more positive. Individuals have a profit-oriented approach. It maximizes their achievements at an individual as well as societal level. In the wake of social development, human differences have been reduced to an extent. People behave more humanely, avoiding racism, fascism, fundamentalism, etc. It promotes nationalism and pluralism with an increase in human rights organizations.

In a developed society, the value orientation is more individual and family-centered. Whatever a person does for the community is based on how much satisfaction he drives from it. Customs and traditions became weaker. Everything from clothes and food to language and style has accelerated.

They have become more continental. Despite religion's exists, religious practices and rites are declining. People have become more rational than before.

- **Political Aspects**

The majority of the countries around the world hold democratic societies. The eradication of the authoritative rule and kinship was the first and most radical form of social change. It brought a sense of nationhood among individuals. Today, liberty is the priority. People enjoy the freedom of speech, choice of profession, religious practices, etc., within their societies.

Social development has removed discrimination among individuals. In a society, every member is equal from whatever caste, creed, or religion he belongs to. They are provided equal opportunities to participate in political, social, and economic affairs. Under the influence of social development, consciousness about non-profit NGOs and welfare organizations has also increased. Individuals are engaged in such healthy activities.

Strategies to Shape Individual's SocialDevelopment

Social development is fundamental at every age. You can still enhance your social capabilities whether you are a child, a youngster, or an adult. It will help you build, maintain and grow more meaningful relationships with family, friends, colleagues,and others.

Here are some strategic ways to work on your social development;

• **Look Inwards**

You might face difficulty in interacting with people. Sometimes, even a general conversation turns into an argument, leading to a relationship break. It indicates the not-so-good level of your social development. If you are also experiencing such challenges, the best approach can be to look inwards.

Pay attention to your emotions, thoughts, and feelings that trigger the negative behavior. When you know the reason causing the problem, it will be easier for you to control it.

- **Fake It till You Make It**

For individuals who find it difficult to talk even in their peer groups, it can be helpful for you to try to appear more social. Whenever you see someone coming to you, say hi and talk about anything you feel like. It might seem weird initially, but you will get the drill with time.

Pretend to be social and talkative among your friends. The more you try talking, no matter how silly it is, the more you can develop into an active being socially.

- **Give Compliments**

Try complimenting your friend when you see your friendship moving to extreme silence. Naturally, people like receiving good comments about themselves. It pleases them and makes others more attentive and closer to you. Hence, giving compliments can let you initiate communication, building into a stronger social bonding.

- **Even Little Things Matter**

People who lack social development should improve little by little. It is about taking baby steps to achieve what you want. You can begin by binding yourself not to think negatively. If you don't feel comfortable talking with your family, try to spend some time practicing that. It might seem difficult at first, but you will enjoy it with time. Such little effort can let you build a strong relationship with your family.

- **Identify & Replace Negative Thoughts**

Having negative perceptions about yourself or social relations can affect your relationships. Sometimes, we self-judge ourselves. When it turns out negative, we criticize and overthink our imperfections. For example, someone who thinks is not deserving of love and attention. Despite others caring for him, he will doubt himself.

The only solution is to identify and replace your negative emotions. Rather than thinking you don't deserve it, remind yourself that you do. Practicing positive affirmations can also bevery helpful in getting rid of negative energy.

- **Improve Your Emotional Intelligence**

At the adult stage of life, some people still don't have the required level of tolerance, patience, and dedication towards their relationship. It is still okay to realize the lacking and improve it for betterment. Try to build yourself emotionally well. You can sustain healthy life-long relationships as long as you can control your emotions.

- **Stay Up to Date**

Keeping yourself aware of current events can assist you in exchanging views. While conversing with your relations generally, you must have something valuable to talk about. Staying up to date allows you to have the necessary informationto share. It helps you engage and communicate, ensuring a meaningful relationship.

- **Join a Support Group**

For individuals facing challenges in social relationships can go for a support group. It provides you with a comforting space to open up. When you interact with individuals, it builds up confidence and speaking ability. It improves your communication skill promoting strong relations.

How to Measure an Individual's SocialDevelopment?

When it comes to measuring social development, there can be many indicators to focus upon. The two most reliable factorsinclude life expectancy (health) and an adult literacy rate (education) to measure on a country level. These country figurescan help measure social development and its progress. However, the effective points to measure an individual's socialdevelopment criteria can be following;

- **Social Competence**

Evaluation of social competence can be a great way to measure someone's social development. If a person finds it challenging to compete socially, he must be lacking. There is a high chance that children who are raised improperly suffer in social competence. They lack confidence in themselves, and criticizing and negative thinking about themselves can also be the reason.

There can be several ways to improve your social competence. Try challenging yourself by participating more socially. Remember winning should not be the goal, but participating is all that matters.

- **Emotional Competence**

A child or an adult can be weak emotionally. This can directly or indirectly affect his relationship with the known and unknown people within a society. You can have an honest review of your emotional capability. How emotionally stable are you? How many times has your dynamic behavior affected your relationship?

Think of the emotional factors that come in between your relations. Knowing your weak points, you can better avoid such situations or feelings. It eventually helps you stay emotionally strong.

- ## Behavior Problems

Individuals who face behavioral disorders like anger, anxiety, intolerance, mood swings, or even mental stress must have reduced social development. Such responses usually are influenced by early childhood experiences. Those who have

- ## Self-Regulation

Self-regulation is all about managing one's behavior to things happening around. However, some socially underdeveloped individuals lack the skill. They find it hard to control their strong negative emotions like frustration or anger. It causes them embarrassment, affecting their social life.

Solutions to self-regulation issues exist. You can opt for self- regulation and management courses or sessions. Therapies and counseling sessions can also be very helpful in this regard.

CHAPTER 15

SOCIAL SKILLS FOR GOOD SOCIAL WELL BEING

Social awkwardness is a part of life. There come times when we don't feel like talking or responding well socially. But to some people, it is what takes all over their social life. Their heartbeat immediately accelerates while interacting with strangers. They would rather disappear or force out a conversation. It all happens to people experiencing social anxiety.

People who lack the skill to socialize comfortably, engage in conversation, or make valuable interactions are **socially inept**. They are either unconfident or anxious enough to misread social cues. For example, when someone makes an offensive joke, it shows his poor social development to interact positively.

Socially inept people typically fear talking to new people. They might be afraid of getting embarrassed. For example, despite being an excellent fit for the company, an individual gets overstressed and cannot respond to the questions in the interview. It can happen due to the lack of engaging ability.

He might feel confused or unable to speak. Have you ever experienced yourself or a friend behaving that way? It is more common among introverts. They try their best to avoid social gatherings and always prefer to stay alone.

Research shows more than 60% of people experience social shyness and anxiety. It is a common fear among individuals, especially in new social settings. You might wonder why even celebrities like Mel Robbins and Jennifer Lawrence have sometimes been socially anxious.

Are you wondering if you are the one among 60% of socially inept? Do you also find it hard to engage socially? Since every individual is unique, there can be several ways you might express your socially inept behavior. You might feel nervous, talk less, make weird expressions, or avoid conversing at all.

Well, here are a few noticeable signs to figure out if you are socially okay or not.

• **Social Nervousness** – You feel anxious or nervous, wanting to end the interaction quickly while communicating with an unknown.

- **The incapability of Being Humorous** – You lack the skill of engaging others through your jokes. People either don't get it or get offended, misunderstanding what you say.

- **Avoiding Social Interactions** – You try to avoid talking to people without purpose, limiting your social exposure.

- **No Conversation Flow** – You can't keep the conversation going while talking to people. You don't know what to say even when you want to speak. It abruptly halts the conversation without reaching a good end.

- **Awkward Silences** – You experience awkwardness causing long silences.

- **Overthinking** – You think a lot about every littlething while communicating. It makes you regret saying certain things. That feeling further encourages you not totalk again.

- **Misreading** – You misread social cues, responding unexpectedly.

- **Awkward Silence** – While talking to people, youbecome silent, not knowing what to say or how to keep it going. Remember, being socially inept never means you have a mental illness. Social awkwardness is more about a person's poor social skills than a personal lacking. Some people are feeling confident in large crowds while shy or anxious in one- to-one meetings. Likewise, there are people who are really goodin small gatherings, but they fear being in public.

Causes of Social Weakness

Social incapability is not a natural deficiency. It usually occurs due to improper social development of a child. When anindividual does not have adequate social exposure in childhood, he ends up staying all on himself. It limits one's opportunity to interact socially. Thus, a person results in becoming socially inept.

There can be several reasons causing social weakness. Someof them are discussed below;

- ### Personality Traits

Some individuals have certain personality traits causing social challenges. It does not mean they lack an ideal personalityor have to be socially inept. They are unique in their own way. Such people can either be introverts or socially inactive. They might not like having many people around. For example, a person is shy by nature. He feels awkward engaging socially. But it does not mean he can't overcome his shyness. With practice and exposure, he can turn into a good social being.

Personal traits are changeable. However, there are some limits because of the underlying aspects of a person's individuality. But almost everyone can improve his social skills. It is just a matter of dedication to build the required level of self-confidence.

- **Not Interested in Social Gatherings**

People become socially inactive when their life is more self-centered. They enjoy staying home, reading books, or treating themselves. It can be the reason they often avoid gatherings, meetups, or outings with friends and family. It is because such individuals are better equipped for loneliness. It does not cause them pain; they are all fine on their own. That is completely normal because not everyone is supposed to be hyperactive or a social adept. But the primary concern is that being so unaware can affect them.

When a person stays busy with himself, he remains uninformed of the community. It can cause him to lag behind others at different stages of life. Therefore, even suchindividuals need to stay connected socially.

- **Lack of Social Development**

Despite humans being natural learners, they need someone to guide them. Many children pick the habit of socializing unconsciously from others. But some children, if not taught properly, keep lacking the skill. It can be the reason why such children develop into socially incapable adults. They don't really know how to interact with strangers.

Learning and adapting things does not have any age limits. Such individuals whose social education has been disrupted for any reason can now resume that. They can join social education classes, sessions or an institute to build up their social skills. Also, teaching social education at educational institutions can be very constructive to facilitate socially inept beings.

- **Uncommon Interests**

A person's social activeness more or less depends on his interests. *How can a person talk about something he is not interested in?* This might be the reason due to which a person feels socially awkward. Let's take an example of a boy who is not interested in cricket. He must have no idea what cricket is orwhat is going on these days. When others discuss, share and engage, he feels super disconnected and not content. The lack of interest and knowledge leads a person to social isolation.

On the other hand, the opposite can also happen. An individual might have different interests than his peers. Some girls in childhood usually don't really like girly things. They love having a short haircut and playing cricket and football rather than what typical girls prefer. Having such distinctive interest and unexpected behavior can minimize social interaction.

Several other factors or deficiencies can also retard an individual's social skills. Children or even adults with, Autism, Social Communication Disorder (SCD), or other conditions can be socially inept to a large extent. Sometimes, even an average active individual feels socially down. It happens due to temporary mood swings, depression or stress.

Social Inadequacies and their causes

Individuals lacking social skills are socially inadequate. Such individuals might face problems in initiating a conversation in a social gathering. They prefer to stay quiet and hide among others. It is majorly due to their social lacking. They don't really know how to fit in a community. However, there can be multiple other reasons behind a person's social inadequacy.

Some of the significant social inadequacies and their causes are discussed below;

- **Social Anxiety**

Social phobia is basically the extreme fear of social settings. Individuals who find it troublesome to talk, meet, and greet new people in social gatherings are socially anxious. Such people might have a fear of being judged by others. They may even want to overcome their anxiety, but feel powerless.

Some people confuse social anxiety with shyness. However, shyness is an entirely different thing. It is usually temporary and lives for a very short term. A person might be shy about meeting his cousin or anyone new first time, but he can overcome the shyness with time. If both continue meeting frequently, they will feel comfortable with each other, and shyness will fade away.

On the other hand, social anxiety remains persistent and deliberate. It continues to affect someone's life for longer. Individuals with social anxiety get bothered in school, at work, and anywhere outside home. They avoid socializing, and it can be due to several reasons.

According to recent research, certain negative experiences and environmental factors contribute the most to causing social anxiety. Bullying, family conflicts, and sexual or emotional abuse can be a few driving factors of social phobia. It can also be adopted from one's family genetically.

- **Social Awkwardness**

Social awkwardness is feeling threatened and doubtful about one's own behavior. It is when a person fears rejection from others. It stimulates an individual's consciousness to either behave in ways to get accepted or stay to himself.

In an attempt to be socially accepted, a person overwhelms. He fails to notice minor social expectations and speaks what he doesn't really mean to. It makes him very uncomfortable, finding almost every social situation difficult to go with.

Social awkwardness usually gets triggered when there is a moral or social transgression. It emerges out of the social tension building through words or body gestures. When an individual tries to reduce the tension, he becomes socially awkward.

- ### Anti-Social Behavior

A behavior involving elements like anger, aggressiveness, hostility, and other negative actions is called an Anti-social behavior. You must have seen people fighting or reacting aggressively to even minor things. Such individuals intentionally or unintentionally threaten their social circle and push them away.

Figuring out the causes of why individuals have anti-social behavior is challenging. There can be varying reasons for each individual case. Medically, it occurs in people with brain disorders like lack of oxygen or nervous irregularities. To other normal individuals, exposure to domestic violence, abusive parents or adults, sexual or emotional distress, drug addiction, or any sort of instability can trigger anti-social behavior.

Social Skills Needed to Achieve SocialWellness

As discussed earlier, social wellness refers to the relationships a person has and how he interacts with others. It encourages the idea of building healthy relationships.

To achieve social wellness, a person needs to have certain social skills. These can be the interpersonal or soft skills to interact and communicate better in a social setting. They help individuals keep up with their personal and professional relations. Some of the primary social skills you need to maintainsocial well-being include the following;

- **Effective Communication**

Communication is the key. The ability to communicate is a core social skill. Every individual needs to transmit his thoughts, ideas, and feelings to other individuals within a social group or community. However, it is only possible through effective communication.

Whether be it bonding with friends, family, or random individuals, it all depends on how better you can communicate.

Poor communication can cause misunderstandings. It can eventually disturb your relations, affecting your social wellness.

- **Conflict Resolution**

Disagreements are a part of life. It is not necessary for everyrelation to flow at the same pace for a lifetime. There come ups and downs in every social setting. But how a person handles and resolves the conflict decides the end outcome.

If you know the skill of agree-to-disagree, you can become a good part of any social gathering. You can play a significant role in dissolving community conflicts and bringing peace to your and everyone else's life. It is ultimately beneficial for your socialwellness.

- **Active Listening**

When it comes to building relations, it is a two-way process. Both the individuals involved in communication need to listen carefully. Therefore, it is very crucial for you to have an active listening ability. You must be patient, attentive, and receptive tothe other person.

Imagine yourself being ignored or overheard in a group of

friends. It must be very displeasing and discouraging. You might not bother to speak or share anything with them the next time. Likewise, you should have an active listening skills to make others feel valued. It makes your relationships worthier and more long-lasting.

- ## Empathy

Being empathetic is a social skill that is very rare. People usually underestimate the emotional connection they can build by understanding someone's feelings. With empathy, you can be there for your relations and let them confide in you. It is natural when we feel more connected to someone who understands the story from our perspective. Similarly, you can also make your relations closer by practicing empathy.

- ## Establishing and Maintaining Personal Relations

Relationships like blood, family, siblings, and relatives are natural. Building relations with friends, colleagues, mates, etc., is a bit difficult. However, what is more testing, yet crucial is sustaining both sorts of relationships.

Family and friends are the ones with whom we spend

quality time. They make us feel comfortable and let us be our true selves. They are the ones whom we call upon in difficult times. Therefore, establishing good relationships is a key to social wellness. People with disturbed or unhealthy relations usually have a terrible quality of life.

Methods & Techniques to ImproveSocial Skills

Each individual is unique and develops a different level of social skills. Some people are proactive and socially adept. They better know how to interact, communicate and make space for themselves. On the other hand, many individuals might be not as good at socializing as others. They are either shy, afraid to interact, or socially anxious. Such social beings typically are so because of their shortcoming in social skills.

If you feel yourself struggling socially, there is no need to worry. Lacking social skills or being poor at it is totally okay. You can try to focus on building up your social skills with time. It might seem challenging, but it is not. Anyone can improve hissocial skills in the following manner;

• **Socialize More**

Do you really want to boost your social skills? If yes, then doing that is simple through socializing more than before. It is evident that only when you will meet people can you have a chance to make a connection and build a relationship. Find ways to engage with surrounding people, initiate conversations and take the lead. It will give you a sense of self-confidence and social strength.

- **Body language**

Regarding socializing, your body language speaks louder than your words. Unless you can show people how attentive and focused you are towards them, you can't let them hook onto you.In a social setting, you must know how to respond to people. Listen to them carefully, make eye contact, and pass on appropriate facial expressions.

- **Observe & Learn from others**

The easiest trick to improve social skills is copying an ideal one. Look around yourself; is there anyone whose social behavior influences you? Once you figure out the person, carefully observe him. It will help you learn how to interact, respond, and behave socially.

Even in some cases, if someone close to you is really good at socializing, you can ask him for help. There is nothing wrong with taking help when you can.

- **Utilize Resources for Social Skills**

Several books, magazines, articles, podcasts, videos, and other content are available. You can search for a particular thing as per your need. Utilize the resources to learn and adapt positive social skills. You better know your own self. Ask yourself what you really need to improve. Are you bad at your body language? Do you lack the ability to listen carefully?

Identify your weak points and utilize resources to improve them.

- **Engage in Social Activities & Communities**

For introverts or socially inept individuals, even ice-breaking can be super hard. If you are one of that types, you can try participating in social activities. It can be a sports club, reading club, community band, meeting group, art and craft circle, or anything that interests you and can be your go-to social place.

Joining such a social activity lets you engage with individuals of similar interests. It is easy for you to interact and build a relationship with them through an activity. For example, if you love reading novels, you can join a reading club. You will definitely love meeting new people there, particularly readers, knowing their favorite authors and exchanging views with them.

- **Ask Questions**

Meeting a new person is fairly challenging. It is because we don't know what to say next. But with a positive socializing mindset, you can take it as an opportunity. Not knowing can even be very helpful in avoiding conversational pauses or social awkwardness. You can simply go on asking more and morequestions.

People love to talk about themselves. By asking questions, you can provide someone a chance to elaborate on himself. Butwhile doing so, make sure to keep your questions open-ended. Itactually helps your conversation flow.

- **Embrace Awkwardness**

While trying to be socially adept, you will have to face awkwardness time and again. It is on you to embrace your fears and overcome your social anxiety. To make it possible, step out of your comfort zone and meet new people. You might feel awkward once, twice, or thrice, but with time, you will see yourself improving.

Embrace social awkwardness as a step towards social adaptation. Rather than considering it a failure, take it productively and stay consistent with your efforts.

At the societal level, the increase in socially inept behaviors can cause adverse effects. It disturbs social harmony, causing social dissatisfaction. In case of any problem, people are supposed to collaborate and find a solution. People lacking social development and have poor socializing skills find it troublesome to work collectively. Therefore, it is high time forevery individual to be socially smart.

The opposite of socially inept is socially adept. A person whohas the skill, competence, and ability to interact well in a socialsetting is **socially adept**. He can better tackle social gatherings and new interactions.

CHAPTER 16

A GUIDE TO BUILDING HEALTHY RELATIONSHIPS

3Cs for Healthy Relationships

Relationships are built on deeper connections and relationships, but their foundations are built on the three crucial characteristics of communication, compromise, and commitment, which are most prevalent in a partnership. Finding the ideal balance between the three can be challenging, but getting through it is what matters most. Here are the three c's of a relationship that you should pay particular attention to.

Communicate

One of the most crucial elements of any relationship, particularly a romantic one, is communication. One of the biggest mistakes couples do is to ignore fights and disagreements rather than discussing them and striving to comprehend one another's viewpoints. Even if walking away from the disagreement and giving yourself some space may help you both forget about it the next day, if you don't learn to grasp what your partner expects from you, you'll continue to run intothese kinds of problems.

Any wholesome relationship must have open communicationas a key element. It's critical to discuss any differences in opinions you and your partner may have when they arise. A healthy relationship requires listening to your partner and taking their advice into consideration. There are occasions when unpleasant topics will come up in a conversation. However, youmay resolve these challenges together if you communicate clearly.

People frequently avoid discussing their issues because theydon't want to get into a disagreement. However, doing so typically only makes things worse. Effective communication with your partner will help you solve any problems that arise andstrengthen your connection.

Compromise

This idea is connected to the previous one in certain ways. Once you've mastered communication, there are instances when compromise is the only option to put an end to a dispute. Some issues can never be resolved if the two of you are wholly unwilling to compromise and entirely committed to your own positions. Learning to occasionally cave in to your mate will require some work. Pick your fights. It may be as basic as deciding which movie you and your date will watch. Don't argue if your girlfriend wants to see the latest girly flick; simply decide that you two will watch an action movie the following week. Clearly, certain circumstances will be considerably more serious, but the same guidelines apply.

In order for a relationship to be stronger, both parties must feel as though they are making a contribution. There will, though, inevitably be problems and disagreements. It's crucial to be able to express yourself freely and to agree to differ in order to keep a relationship healthy. Because of this, decisions may be made freely and without undue pressure for either party. By making a compromise, you communicate to your partner that you value the union enough to try to resolve any differences that may arise.

Commitment

It's harder said than done to communicate and compromise with your significant other. You might go through them and consider, "No issue. I am capable of doing that." When it comes down to it, though, it will require work from both you and your partner. It will eventually fail if you aren't entirely devoted to mending your tense connection. You will both need to concentrate on exercising patience and paying close attention to your partner's needs if you want your relationship to succeed.

A relationship is much simpler to end without commitment. In a committed relationship, promises are crucial because they assist both parties to stay accountable and remind them of the reasons they started dating in the first place. Although staying committed to one another makes it much easier, staying together through good times and bad is not always simple.

If you want your relationship to last, you both need to be emotionally and physically devoted to one another. Lack of commitment frequently results in infidelity, mistrust, and ultimately a breakup. By committing to your partner, you are showing them that you respect their contribution to your life and that you are in it for the long run.

It is possible to make your relationship work if you both agree that taking the time to mend it is worthwhile and you are both committed to doing so. Sometimes just one person needs to start the process of counseling in order for the relationship to transform. You should be headed in the right direction toward a closer, more loving relationship if you stop ignoring your disputes and start learning to occasionally compromise. It's all about working together and making each other feel cherished, loved, and respected.

Improving Communication Skills is Key to Any Relationship

A good partnership requires effective communication, which is a crucial component of all relationships. All relationships have their ups and downs, but having a good communication style can help you deal with disagreements and forge a stronger, healthier relationship.

What is Communication?

The transmission of information from one location to another is the definition of communication. In a relationship, communication enables you to express to the other person your feelings and requirements. Communicating not only enables you to get what you need but also strengthens the bond between you and your partner.

Clear Communication in A Relationship

Chat with one another. You cannot read your partner's mind, no matter how well you know and love each other. To prevent misconceptions that can lead to hurt, rage, resentment, or confusion, we must speak clearly.

Relationships require two people, each of whom has unique communication needs and preferences. Finding a communication strategy that works for a couple's relationship is essential. Effective communication requires effort and hardwork. There will never be an ideal time for communication.

When speaking with your partner, be explicit so that your point is accepted and comprehended. Verify that you have understood all your spouse has said.

Benefits of Effective Communication in Relationships

The Gottman Institute's founder, clinical psychologist Dr. John Gottman, claims that a couple's communication style frequently indicates how successful a relationship will be. Several ways that effective communication might improve yourrelationship are as follows:

• It can reduce dwell time: Effective communication enables people to express their worries and find more constructive solutions to them rather thanstewing over unfavorable emotions.

• It promotes intimacy: Establishing a strong

emotional bond with another person calls for a reciprocal exchange of information about yourself in exchange for their perspective. Talking about your experiences, views, values, opinions, and expectations is a part of this reciprocal self-disclosure. You both must be able to communicate effectively for this connection to befostered and allowed to develop over time.

• Conflict in every relationship eventually arises and needs to be reduced or resolved. However, you can settle disputes more quickly when you are able to discuss your issues in an open and honest manner. You may discuss your issues and take action to strengthen your relationship rather than becoming sucked into a loop of misunderstandings, wounded feelings, and emotionalstrife.

Communication Is Not a Cure-All

While it has long been believed that better communication is the best way to start improving a relationship, new research indicates that the solution may not be as straightforward as it first appears.

According to research reported in the Journal of Marriage and Family, while there is unquestionably a link between effective communication and relationship happiness, strong communication doesn't by itself guarantee that you'll be happy in your relationships.

There is a wealth of evidence demonstrating that good communication skills improve relationships and well-being in a variety of ways, even while it implies that communicating effectively isn't a guarantee for a successful relationship.

One method to develop a good, supportive relationship with your partner is through effective communication. Both of you are more likely to feel respected and cared for when you actively listen to and respond to your partner (and they do the same for you).

For instance, a study discovered that people are more likely to sleep well when they feel their partner values them. Finally, having relationships that make you feel more appreciated, optimistic, and content might be good for your general well- being.

Communication Effectiveness Characteristics

What do professionals mean when they refer to "excellent communication"? Are you and your partner on the same page or are there any warning signals that your relationship may be having issues?

First, it's critical to consider what exactly we mean by communication. It appears that it has to do with the words that individuals use to communicate with one another. However, it can also involve nonverbal cues like tone of voice, body language, and other nonverbal means of communication. What you don't say often has just as much, if not more, impact thanwhat you do.

The following are some characteristics of relationships whencommunication is effective:

•   Active listening entails participating in the conversation, paying close attention, and summarizing what has been said. It also entails refraining from passing judgment and seeking clarification when necessary.

•   Not personalizing issues: People who are effective at communicating in relationships don't make their partner's behavior personally. Instead, they concentrate on the problem and it's solutions.

•   Using "I" statements: In interpersonal situations, "I" remarks can be useful. Try using an I-statement instead of saying, "You never clean up after yourself," such as, "I feel uncomfortable when there is clutterbuilding up around the house."

•   Kindness: Being kind to others is crucial becauseit makes them feel valued and understood.

•   Being present: It's crucial to be completely in themoment when speaking with your partner. Distractions from the outside world, even technological ones like your phone, can cause a breakdown in communicationand connection.

•   Accepting the other person even if you don't agree with them is an important part of healthy communication. When you and your spouse are able to communicate effectively, you may acknowledge that individuals have the right to feel what they are feeling, even if those sentiments and reactions are different from your own.

How to Communicate More Effectively

There are ways to strengthen your connection if you believe that a lack of clear communication is harming your relationship.

Keep Your Attachment Style in Mind

Consider how your communication style may be impacted by your attachment style. Your distinctive interpersonal behavioral patterns are known as your attachment styles. Your early attachment style, which develops during childhood as a result of your interactions with caregivers, can still have an impact on how you act and react in love relationships as an adult.

If you have an uneasy attachment style, you can be more prone to using avoidant or anxious communication techniques. You can get hints into what you might need to improve on by recognizing how your attachment style impacts how you engage with your spouse (and how their style affects how they interact with you).

Being Present

Reduce distractions and concentrate on being totally present while communicating to ensure that both of you are listening and comprehending. Setting aside time each day to genuinely pay attention to one another and discuss the day's happenings as well as any worries you may have may be necessary for this.

Limiting your usage of devices during specific periods of theday, such as meals or before bed, can be a terrific way to concentrate on your partner without being distracted by other things.

Use "I" statements.

Communication issues can occasionally be greatly impactedby the way you talk to each other. Arguments can easily devolveinto arguments about who is "correct" or who gets the final word if you and your opponent are only disputing the facts and not your feelings.

By employing this style of statement, you and your partner can focus on the feelings underlying some of the problems you are concerned about, makingconversations sound lessaccusatory or blaming.

Stay Away from Negative Communication Styles

When you feel the want to rant, ignore your partner, or use passive-aggressive tactics, stop and think about how your behavior will damage your relationship. Since many of these patterns were established during childhood, changing them isn'talways simple, but becoming more conscious of them can help you begin to replace these negative behaviors with healthier, more constructive routines.

Put Your Relationship First

Despite its importance, research indicates that effective communication is only one of several aspects that affect the success, longevity, and pleasure of partnerships.

In fact, it appears that communication between you and your partner may be predicted by your relationship satisfaction. People are more likely to be honest and open with one another about their ideas, feelings, worries, and difficulties when they are more content in their relationship.

Identifying Abuse in a Relationship

Emotional Abuse: What Is It?

The act of controlling someone else emotionally by criticizing, humiliating, shaming, blaming, or otherwise manipulating them is known as emotional abuse. Mental or emotional abuse can happen in any connection, including those with friends, family, and coworkers, despite being more often indating and married partnerships.

The main objective of emotional abuse is to isolate, discredit, and silence the other person in order to exert control over them. One of the most difficult types of abuse to spot because it can be sneaky and subtle. It can, however, also be overt and deceptive.

Emotional abuse can undermine your self-esteem in either case, and you can start to question your views and reality. Finally, you might feel confined. People who have experienced emotional abuse are frequently too hurt to remain in the relationship but also too terrified to abandon it. So, until something is done, the cycle will continue.

Emotional Abuse Warning Signs

The signs of emotional abuse are numerous. Remember that your connection with your partner, parent, coworker, or friend is still emotionally abusive even if they only engage in a small number of these behaviors rather than all of them.

Also keep in mind that emotional abuse is frequently imperceptible while you think about your relationship. As a result, it may be very challenging to spot the warning indications. Think about how your interactions make you feel if you are having problems determining whether your relationship is abusive.

Additionally, avoid rationalizing the other person's actions by telling yourself "it's not that bad." Everyone, including you, needs to be treated with respect and kindness. You can break the pattern of emotional abuse by realizing this.

Unrealistic Expectations

If someone has unreasonable expectations for you, that may be an indication of emotional abuse. Several instances of this are:

- Putting forth irrational demands

- Requiring you to put everything else aside in order to attend to their needs

- Requesting that you spend all of your time with them

- Being unsatisfied despite your best efforts and sacrifices

- Criticizing you for failing to do things to their expectations

- Expecting you to express what they think (i.e., you are not permitted to have a different opinion)

- Demanding that when describing things that distress you, you give precise dates and times (and whenyou cannot do this, they may dismiss the event as if it never happened)

Invalidates You

If they invalidate you, they can be engaging in emotionalabuse. An illustration of invalidation is:

- Denying, ignoring, or manipulating your reality or your perceptions

- Attempting to determine how you should feel in order to avoid acknowledging your sensations

- Demanding constant explanations of your feelings calling you "too sensitive," "too emotional," or "crazy"
- Refusing to respect or accept your thoughts as legitimate

- Rejecting your demands, desires, and needs as absurd or unjustified

- Sayings like "you're blowing this out of proportion" or "you exaggerate" that imply your senses are off or that you cannot be trusted.

- If you voice your demands or needs, people may accuse you of being egotistical, dependent, or materialistic (the expectation is that you should not haveany wants or needs)

- **Causes Chaos**

- People who abuse emotions also have a tendency to stir uptrouble. These are some instances of this warning sign:

- Launching debates merely for the sake of debate

- Making claims that are unclear and incoherent (sometimes called "crazy-making")

- Experiencing abrupt mood shifts or emotional outbursts
- Critiquing your work, attire, hair, and other aspects

- Acting in such an unpredictable and chaotic manner that you feel as though you are "stepping on eggshells"

Emotionally Blackmailing

Emotional abuse is evident if someone tries to control youremotions against you. Emotional blackmail instances include:

- Giving you a guilt trip; manipulating and influencing you by inducing guilt

- Using your fears, values, compassion, or other sensitive areas to manipulate you or the circumstance by humiliating you in public or privately

- Highlighting or exaggerating your weaknesses to divert attention or avoid accepting responsibility for theirown poor decisions or errors

- Denying or exaggerating the occurrence of an event

- Denying you love or giving you the silent treatment as a form of punishment

Acts Superior

Emotionally abusive individuals frequently display arrogance and entitlement. When evaluating whether the individual in your life demonstrates this symptom of emotionalabuse, look for the following things:

- Treating you as if you're less than

- Accusing you of their errors and failings

- Doubting everything you say and making aneffort to disprove you

- Joking around about you

- Claiming that your beliefs, principles, and way of thinking are absurd, illogical, or "do not make sense"

- Being patronizing or condescending to you

- Joking around with you in a sarcastic manner

- Acting as if they are always correct, have better knowledge than you, and are intelligent

Isolates and Controls You

People that abuse your emotions will try to dominate and isolate you. These are a few instances of this type of emotional abuse:

- Limiting your social interactions with everyone,

319

even your relatives and friends

- Keeping an eye on you online, including through email, social media, and SMS messaging

- Accusing you of infidelity and expressing resentment toward other people's relationships

- Take or conceal your car keys.

- Need to always know where you are or utilizing GPS to follow your every move

- Treating you like a tool or a piece of property

- Making fun of or critiquing your friends, family, and coworkers

- Using envy and jealousy to prevent you from being with others and to serve as a display of love

- Forcing you to spend every moment together
- In charge of the finances

Dealing with Emotional Abuse

Recognizing the abuse is the first step in dealing with an emotionally abusive relationship. It is crucial to first and foremost acknowledge any instances of emotional abuse in yourrelationship if you can.

You may regain control of your life by being honest about what you are going through. Here are seven other methods you may do right away to take back control of your life.

Put your needs first.

Put yourself first when it comes to your physical and mental wellbeing. Put an end to trying to appease the abuser. Attend to your requirements. Make a decision that will encourage optimistic thinking and self-affirmation.

Additionally, make sure you get enough sleep and eat nutritious foods. You may deal with the daily challenges of emotional abuse with the help of these easy self-care techniques.

Create Boundaries

Tell the abusive person firmly that you will no longer tolerate their yelling, name-calling, insulting, rudeness, etc. Afterward, explain what will occur if they decide to engage in this conduct.

Tell them, for instance, that the conversation will end and youwill leave the room if they insult you or call you names.

The secret is to stick to your bounds. The other person will understand that their emotional abuse will not be permitted as aresult of this.

Don't Blame Yourself Ever Again

You could think there is something seriously wrong with youif you've been in an emotionally abusive relationship for a while. But the issue is not with you. Abuse involves a decision. Stop blaming yourself for things that are out of your control.

Understand You Can't Fix Them

You will never be able to change an emotionally abusive person by acting differently or by changing who you are, no matter how hard you try. A person who is abusive chooses to actin an abusive manner.

Avoid Interacting

Avoid interacting with someone who is abusive. In other words, do not try to justify yourself, allay their concerns, or apologize for something you did not do if an abuser tries to create an argument with you, insults you, makes demands of you, or becomes enraged with jealousy.

If you can, just leave the matter alone. If you interact with an abuser, you will only experience more suffering and violence. You won't be able to make things right in their eyes, no matter how hard you try.

Create a Support System

Even though it may be difficult, speaking up might be helpful if you are experiencing emotional abuse. Discuss your feelings with a close friend, a member of your family, or a counselor. Spend as much time as you can away from the abusive individual and with the people who love and support you.

You'll feel less alone and isolated thanks to this group of wholesome pals and confidantes. Additionally, they have the ability to bring truth into your life and aid with perspective- setting.

Prepare an Exit Strategy

You cannot stay in an abusive relationship indefinitely if yourpartner has no intention of improving or changing their bad habits. It will eventually have an adverse effect on your mental and physical health.

You might need to take action to break up with the person,

depending on your circumstances. Every circumstance is unique. Therefore, talk about your thoughts and ideas with a close friend, member of your family, or counselor. In addition to having negative long-term repercussions, emotional abuse can also serve as a prelude to physical abuse and other forms of violence.

Also keep in mind that when the victim of the abuse decidesto leave, the abuse frequently gets worse. Therefore, make sure that you have a safety plan in place in case the abuse intensifies.

Keeping Your Relationship Alive

Your relationship with your significant other is and ought to be your top priority in life. But because of the stress of daily life, you take your relationship for granted. Before you realize it, neither your demands nor those of your partner is satisfied.

But you're not to blame. We are unaware that maintaining our connections requires work. When things aren't going well, sure, we'll run to the therapist. How do long-term spouses keep the spark alive and the fire blazing in their relationship?

Express Your Needs

It's crucial that you set aside time when challenging situations arise so that everyone has a chance to express their views. A conversation where both of you have a say and agree to constructively discuss and work through your issues, both aloneand together.

It's crucial to set out all pertinent information and emotions so that you can build a solid communication foundation. You want your spouse to be aware of and considerate of your needs, but you can only do this by having an honest conversation. It's crucial to express your demands in order to maintain a healthy connection.

Plan Intimate Dates

It is advisable for you and your partner to work on scheduling weekly intimacy dates into your busy schedules and finding time for physical closeness. Intimacy dates go beyond simple conversation and physical contact to promote physical connection. It's not necessary for intimacy dates to result in physical contact. It's crucial to prepare for them and choose settings with no outside distractions. The intimacy dates are intended to maintain your sexual relationship.

Don't Hold Your Partner Liable

When your physical and emotional demands are not addressed, frustration sets in. Often, harmful feelings like blame and shame harm the relationship instead of helping the two of you work as a team to find the root of intimacy issues. It is simpler to blame your partner than to consider your own involvement in the issue. Reclaiming your enthusiasm for one another is much more difficult when you start placing blame on one another. Keep in mind that intimacy is a shared experience between couples, not between people.

Embrace Intimacy

Making your partner feel desirable is crucial. There are people struggling to initiate physical affection and intimacy withtheir relationships, either out of unresolved rage or fear ofrejection. The issue with this is that it keeps them from investing time and effort in this crucial aspect of their relationship. You want to ensure that your spouse feels desired by you in order tokeep the connection "alive." Your partner will be reminded of your attraction to them and desire to feel close to them when you start an intimate relationship.

CHAPTER 17

NEW WORLD, NEW CHALLENGES

COVID-19 and Its Impact

The COVID-19 epidemic has caused a shocking loss of life on a global scale and poses an unprecedented threat to food systems, public health, and the workplace. The pandemic has had a devastating impact on the economy and society. Tens of millions of people face the possibility of living in abject poverty, and the number of undernourished people—which is currently estimated to be close to 690 million—could rise by as many as 132 million by the end of the year.

Numerous businesses are in danger of dying out. The livelihoods of over half of the 3.3 billion workers worldwide are in jeopardy. Workers in the informal economy are particularly vulnerable because the majority do not have access to social safety, high-quality healthcare, or productive assets. Many people are unable to provide for themselves and their families during lockdowns because they lack the means of earning a living. For the majority, going without food means eating less unhealthily or, at best, not eating at all.

The epidemic has been having an impact on the whole food system and exposed its vulnerability. Border closures, trade restrictions, and confinement measures have made it difficult for farmers to access markets, including to buy inputs and sell theirproduce, and for agricultural workers to harvest crops. As a result, domestic and global food supply chains have been disrupted, and the availability of a variety of safe, healthy diets has decreased. The pandemic has devastated jobs and placed millions of livelihoods in jeopardy. Millions of women's and men's food security and nutrition are at risk as breadwinners losetheir jobs, get sick, or pass away; those in low-income nations, especially the most marginalized populations, such as small- scale farmers and indigenous peoples, are severely hurt.

While helping to feed the globe, millions of paid and unpaidagricultural laborers often experience high levels of working poverty, starvation, and bad health, as well as a lack of safety and labor protections as well as various forms of abuse. Due to their poor and inconsistent salaries and a lack of social assistance, many of them are motivated to continue working, frequently in hazardous situations, putting their families and themselves at further risk. Additionally, when facing income losses, individuals could turn to harmful coping mechanisms such as asset distress sales, predatory lending, or child labor. Migrant agricultural laborers are especially vulnerable because they suffer dangers in their transportation, employment, and living situations and find it difficult to access government-sponsored support programs. To save lives and safeguard the public's health, people's livelihoods, and food security, it will be essential to ensure the safety and health of all agri-food workers, from primary farmers to those involved in food processing, transport, and retail, including street food sellers.

Food security, public health, employment, and labor issues, especially worker health and safety, come together in the COVID-19 situation. The human aspect of the issue must be addressed by upholding workplace safety and health standards, ensuring access to good employment, and protecting workers' rights across all sectors of the economy. Extending social protection toward universal health coverage and providing economic support for those most impacted should be part of an immediate and focused effort to save lives and livelihoods. These people include youth, older workers, and migrants who work in low-paying, poorly protected, and unorganized sectors of the economy. Women's circumstances require special consideration because they predominate in low-paying jobs and caregiving responsibilities. Cash transfers, child allowances, nutritious school lunches, initiatives to provide shelter and food aid, help for the retention and recovery of jobs, and financial assistance for businesses, including micro, small, and medium- sized ones, are all important types of support. Governments must collaborate closely with employers and employees when developing and implementing such policies. Particularly vulnerable to the consequences of COVID-19 are those that are currently dealing with humanitarian crises or emergencies. It is crucial to react to the pandemic quickly while making sure that relief and rehabilitation aid reaches those who need it the most.

The globe needs to unite in solidarity and support those who are most in need, especially in the growing and developing world. Only by working together will we be able to combat the pandemic's interconnected health, social, and economic effects and stop it from worsening into a protracted humanitarian and food security crisis that could undo development progress that has already been made.

As stated in the UN Secretary-Policy General's Brief, we must seize this chance to rebuild more effectively. We are committed to using our knowledge and experience to assist nations in their efforts to implement crisis response plans and realize the Sustainable Development Goals. The health and agri- food industries are confronting challenges that require the development of long-term, sustainable policies. Priority should be given to tackling the root causes of food security and malnutrition, combating rural poverty, particularly by creating more and better jobs in the rural economy, extending social protection to everyone, facilitating safe migration routes, and promoting the formalization of the informal economy.

Impact of COVID-19 on Mental Health

The COVID-19 pandemic, one of the most significant globalcatastrophes in centuries, has had significant and far-reaching effects on health systems, economics, and civilizations. Numerous people have perished or lost their jobs. Communities and families have become strained and fractured. Young people have been denied the opportunity to learn and interact with others. Companies have filed for bankruptcy. Millions of individuals are now living in poverty.

The mental health of people has been significantly impacted as a result of these health, social, and economic effects. Many of us experienced increased anxiety, but for some COVID-19 has precipitated or exacerbated much more severe mental health issues. Many people have expressed psychological suffering as well as signs of post-traumatic stress disorder, anxiety, or despair. Additionally, there have been alarming indications of a wider prevalence of suicide ideas and actions, even in the healthcare industry.

Some people groups have been impacted significantly more than others. Young people have been left exposed to social isolation and disconnection as a result of prolonged school and university closures. These conditions can exacerbate emotions of worry, uncertainty, and loneliness and result in emotional and behavioral disorders. Being forced to stay at home may have increased the chance of familial stress or abuse, which are risk factors for mental health issues, for some kids and teenagers. Women have also suffered more stress at home; according to one fast evaluation, 45% of women experienced violence during the first year of the pandemic, either directly or indirectly.

Mental health services have been severely disrupted while mental health needs have increased. Early in the epidemic, when personnel and infrastructure were frequently redeployed to COVID-19 relief, this was particularly true.

Social restrictions at the time also made it difficult for people to receive care. And in many instances, lack of information and disinformation about the virus fueled people's anxieties and worries, preventing them from getting medical attention.

Fear and isolation

Stress and anxiety have been brought on by the worry of catching SARS-CoV-2, the virus that causes COVID-19, as well as worries about the impact on the economy.

Due to the increased strain, front-line employees, notably medical professionals, have developed chronic stress and burnout.

Lee Chambers, a psychologist and the creator of Essentials Workplace Wellbeing, claims that frequent lockdowns, physical distance, and fear of infection have all exacerbated isolation, loneliness, and anxiety and are "huge catalysts" for mental health problems.

Worldwide increases in mental health issues

According to a 2019 study published in The Lancet, 12.5% of the world's population will experience mental health issues at some point in their lives. The WHO announced in March 2022 that in the first year of the epidemic, anxiety and despair soared by 25% globally.

Lee Chambers has seen evidence of this: "If I'm honest, from my perspective, the incidence of everything [mental health-related] has increased. […] It has been amplified for people who are already suffering from certain conditions. They've found less access to services and challenges in managing their everyday existence."

He added: "One thing that continually got flagged was new incidences. People who had never previously identified as having any mental health condition had actually disclosed […] or, in surveys, said they were struggling significantly. That is interesting, as it shows the impact is reaching beyond those who have already impacted pre-[COVID-19]."

Early impact

The pandemic's start appears to have had the most effect on mental health. Increasing mental health concerns have been noted recently in numerous European nations, according to a report from the European Parliament Research Service.

In Italy, eight out of ten people said they needed psychological assistance, while in the Netherlands, more than athird of people said they felt anxious.

Similar tendencies become obvious in the United States. In apoll of individuals between the ages of 18 and 35, 80% of participants reported having substantial depressive symptoms, while 61% said they had moderate to severe anxiety.

The National Institute of Mental Health revealed in April 2021 that rates for suicidal ideation, substance abuse, stress- related symptoms, and anxiety were nearly twice as high as anticipated before the epidemic.

The Centers for Disease Control and Prevention (CDC) reports that suicide rates have decreased somewhat, dispelling worries that they would increase.

Who suffers the most?

Younger respondents and those who had already been diagnosed with mental illness reported worse mental health during the early months of the epidemic, according to an analysis of more than 200,000 persons in northern Europe. But these populations are not the only ones who experience mental health problems.

Young people may be less likely to become infected with

SARS-CoV-2, but the pandemic's impacts still affect them. Education, employment, and social connections have all suffered setbacks.

The International Labor Organization stated in August 2020 that "the pandemic's impact on young people is systematic, deep,and disproportionate."

According to a number of studies, the pandemic was associated with greater rates of depression and post-traumatic stress disorder (PTSD) symptoms in students.

In the forefront

The demands on medical personnel have been great. In addition to having to deal with the demands of their changing roles throughout the pandemic, they also had to deal with ongoing exposure to SARS-CoV-2, which unavoidably had animpact on their mental health.

In a meta-analysis of research looking at how the pandemic affected healthcare workers' mental health, it was discovered that stress, anxiety, and depression were the most commonconditions. In addition to burnout, insomnia, infection anxiety, and suicidal thoughts, many healthcare personnel complained.

Not just hospital staff members who work with COVID-19 patients have been impacted. Primary care physicians worldwide experience significant levels of work-related stress, anxiety, and burnout, according to a global assessment of studies that was published in the British Journal of General Practice.

This could have the unsettling effect of leading to many doctors quitting their careers. According to a recent study by the British Medical Association, 21% of respondents were thinking about leaving the NHS and 25% were thinking about taking a career sabbatical as a result of the stress of dealing with the pandemic.

Self-care strategies

Self-care techniques can help you take control of your life and are beneficial for both your physical and mental health. To improve your mental health, look after your body, mind, andrelationships with others.

Take good care of yourself.

Be aware of your bodily well-being: Get adequate rest. Set a regular schedule for bedtime and wakeup. Even if you're staying at home, try to maintain your usual sleeping and wakinghours.

Engage in routine physical activity: Regular exercise and physical activity can lower anxiety and elevate mood. Look for a movement-based activity, like dance or an exercise app. Go outside, perhaps to your backyard or a nearby nature trail.

Healthy eating: Pick a diet that is well-balanced. Refined sugar and junk food should be limited. Limit your caffeine intake because it can make stress, anxiety, and sleep issues worse.

Avoid using alcohol, tobacco, and drugs. You already have an increased risk of lung illness if you smoke or vape. Your risk goes up much worse because COVID-19 damages the lungs. Alcohol can make problems worse and make it harder for you to cope. To cope, stay away from narcotics unless your doctor has recommended them.

Reduce your screen time. Turn off electronics occasionally throughout the day, ideally between 30 and 60 minutes before going to bed. Reduce the amount of time you spend in front of screens, including those on your phone, tablet, computer, and television.

Unwind and revitalize. Schedule some alone time. Even a short period of solitude can be reviving, calm your thoughts, and lessen worry. Practices like deep breathing, tai chi, yoga, mindfulness, or meditation are beneficial to a lot of people. Whatever calms you down, do it: take a bubble bath, listen to music, read a book, or both. Choose a method that works for youand use it frequently.

Maintain your mental health.

Reduce the causes of stress

Maintain your daily regimen: Your mental health will benefit from maintaining a consistent daily schedule. Maintain consistent mealtimes, showering and getting dressed routines, job or study schedules, and exercise plans in addition to adheringto a regular nighttime routine. Make time for your favorite pastimes as well. You may feel more in control as a result of thispredictability.

Limit your news media exposure. Fears about COVID-19 can increase if there is constant reporting about the illness in all forms of media. Use social media in moderation to avoid being exposed to rumors and misleading information. Limit your exposure to other news sources as well, but stay up with local and national guidelines. Look for trustworthy sources, including the U.S. the World Health Organization (WHO) and the Centers for Disease Control and Prevention (CDC) (WHO).

Keep active. You can break the loop of unfavorable thoughts that feed anxiety and despair by engaging in constructive diversions. Take advantage of pastimes you can perform at home, such as reading, journaling, crafting, playing games, or cooking. Or decide on a new undertaking or organize that closet you said you'd do. An effective coping mechanism for anxiety is to take constructive action.

Think only good things. Instead of obsessing on how miserable you feel, make the decision to pay attention to the good things in your life. Consider beginning each day by making a gratitude list. Try to retain a positive outlook, work at accepting changes as they come, and keep concerns in perspective.

Use your spirituality or moral compass as a source of strength. A belief system that you take support from might give you solace in trying and uncertain circumstances.

Place priorities. Don't let making a life-changing list of things to accomplish while you're home overwhelm you.

Everyday, make attainable goals and plan the steps you can take to achieve them. No matter how modest, give yourself credit for every step you take in the correct path. additionally, acknowledge that some days will be more favorable than others.

Relate to others

Develop assistance and bolsterconnections:
Identify connections. Avoid social isolation if you work remotely from home or must distance yourself from people for a while owing to COVID-19. Make time each day to communicate virtually via email, texts, phone calls, or video chats. Ask your coworkers how they're dealing if you're working remotely from home, and offer your own coping mechanisms. Enjoy talking to people in your home on the internet and socializing.

When interacting with people in person if you aren't fully immunized, think outside the box and practice safety. Consider going for walks, having conversations in the driveway, and otheroutside activities, or wearing a mask for interior activities.

If you are fully immunized, you can more safely resume a

variety of indoor and outdoor activities, including getting together with friends and family, that you might not have been able to do due to the epidemic.

However, the CDC advises wearing a mask indoors or outdoors in crowded locations or in close contact with unvaccinated persons if you live in a region where there have been a lot of new COVID-19 cases in the past week. Outdoor activities with lots of space between you and other participants represent a reduced risk of COVID-19 viral transmission for unvaccinated individuals than do interior activities.

Give back to others. Helping those in your neighborhood can give you purpose. A great method to help ourselves is to helpothers. Check on your friends, relatives, and neighbors, especially the elderly, by email, text, or phone, for instance. Ask if there is anything needed, such as groceries or a prescription picked up, if you know someone who is unable to leave their home.

Support a friend or member of your family. Plan strategies to stay in touch if a friend or family member needs to be quarantined at home or in a hospital because of COVID-19. This could be done, for instance, by writing a note to make someone's day brighter or using a phone or technological device.

CHAPTER 18

MINDFULNESS AND WELL-BEING

In the relentless hustle and bustle of modern life, with its constant notifications and unending to-do lists, we often find ourselves swept up in the currents of our thoughts and emotions. But amidst the chaos, a beacon of calm emerges, an ancient practice that offers a sanctuary for our restless minds: Mindfulness. Let's dive deep into understanding mindfulness and its undeniable connection to well-being.

The Essence of Mindfulness

Being fully present is the foundation of mindfulness. It's the delicate skill of impartially examining our thoughts, feelings, physical sensations, and external surroundings. Instead of replaying the past or anticipating the future, mindfulness anchors us in the here and now.

Historical Roots of Mindfulness

Tracing its origins to Buddhist meditation, mindfulness has been practiced for millennia. However, its benefits are not just restricted to spiritual realms. Over the past few decades, Western psychology has integrated mindfulness techniques, highlighting its profound impact on mental health and overall well-being.

The Mind-Body Connection

Our thoughts, emotions, and physical sensations are intricately intertwined. A worrisome idea can quicken our heartbeat, while a moment of joy can lighten our steps. Through mindfulness, we become keenly aware of these connections. By observing our thoughts without being entangled in them, we can better navigate our emotional landscape and its subsequent impact on our bodies.

The Benefits of Mindfulness for Well-being

1. **Reduces Stress:** Regular mindfulness reduces the body's stress hormones, fostering a sense of calm even in turbulent situations.

2. **Enhances Emotional**

Regulation: By being present with our emotions without judgment, we can process and respond to them more rationally.

3. **Improves Focus:** Mindfulness hones our attention, allowing us to concentrate on tasks without distractions.

4.   **Fosters Empathy:** As we become more attuned to our emotions, our capacity to understand and resonate with others' feelings expands.

5.   **Boosts Creativity:** With a clear, focused mind, new and innovative ideas flow more freely.

6.   **Enhances Sleep Quality:** Mindful relaxation techniques can ease the mind, leading to deeper, more restful sleep.

7.   **Supports Physical Health:** From lowering blood pressure to bolstering the immune system, the benefits of mindfulness cascade throughout the body.

Mindfulness in Everyday Life

You don't need to spend hours in meditation to cultivate mindfulness. Here are simple ways to incorporate it into your daily routine:

Mindful Eating: Savor each bite. Be mindful of the flavors, textures, and scents of your meal. This not only enhances your dining experience but also promotes better digestion.

Mindful Walking: Instead of rushing from point A to B,

walk intentionally. Feel the ground beneath your feet, notice the rhythm of your breath, and soak in your environment.

Mindful Breathing: Focus solely on your breath for a few moments each day. This anchors your mind and can be especially beneficial when feeling overwhelmed.

Challenges in Cultivating Mindfulness

As simple as it sounds, mindfulness can be challenging, especially for beginners. Our minds are conditioned to be in a state of constant chatter. However, it's essential to remember that the goal isn't to eliminate thoughts but to observe them without judgment. With time and practice, the process becomes more intuitive.

Technological Aids for Mindfulness

The digital age, often blamed for dwindling attention spans, also offers tools to aid our mindfulness journey. Numerous apps provide guided meditations, breathing exercises, and daily mindfulness prompts to keep you grounded.

The Ripple Effects of Mindfulness

When we are mindful, we are not just improving our well-being. The calm and clarity that comes with mindfulness ripple outwards, positively affecting our relationships and interactions. A conscious individual listens more intently, responds more thoughtfully, and emanates an aura of tranquility that can be contagious.

Mindfulness is more than just a trend or buzzword; it's a way of life. By embracing the present moment, we can navigate the complexities of life with grace and poise. As we foster this heightened awareness, we realize that well-being is about physical health and nurturing a mind at peace, regardless of external circumstances. Through mindfulness, we don't just exist; we thrive.

Benefits of Practicing Mindfulness for Physical and Mental Health

At the convergence of ancient wisdom and modern science lies a practice as simple as it is profound: Mindfulness. More than just a buzzword, mindfulness offers a treasure trove of benefits for our minds and bodies. Let's embark on a journey to uncover the transformative power of mindfulness and how it can enhance our physical and mental well-being.

Mindfulness

Before diving into its benefits, it's crucial to define mindfulness. In its simplest form, mindfulness is wholly present in the current moment. It's about experiencing life as it unfolds without being colored by past regrets or future anxieties. It's the art of observation without judgment.

Physical Health Benefits of Mindfulness

1. **Boosts Immune Function:** Regular mindfulness practices, like meditation, have been linked to improved immune system function. A more robust immune system means fewer illnesses and a faster recovery when we fall sick.

2. **Reduces Chronic Pain:** Mindfulness meditation has been used as a supplementary treatment to treat chronic pain. Many individuals report decreased pain levels and an increased ability to cope with discomfort by focusing on the present.

3. **Improves Sleep:** Mindfulness practices can improve sleep quality by reducing the mental clutter that often keeps us awake. Deep, restorative sleep is crucial for physical health, from cellular repair to energy restoration.

4.   **Lowers Blood Pressure:** Mindfulness can activate the body's relaxation response, reducing blood pressure. This is immensely beneficial for heart health and overall longevity.

5.   **Promotes Healthy Eating:** Mindful eating – savoring each bite, recognizing when you're full, and truly enjoying your food – can help maintain a healthy weight and improve digestion.

Mental Health Benefits of Mindfulness

1.   **Alleviates Symptoms of Depression and Anxiety:** Regular mindfulness practice can change the structure and function of the brain in ways that are consistent with better emotional health. For many, this leads to reduced symptoms of depression and anxiety.

2.   **Increases Attention and Focus:** In an era of constant distractions, the ability to focus is invaluable. Mindfulness hones our attention, making it easier to concentrate on tasks without our minds wandering.

3.   **Boosts Emotional Regulation:** Mindfulness equips us with the tools to observe our emotions without getting swept up, resulting in improved mood regulation and emotional resilience.

4. **Fosters a Positive Mindset:** Regular mindfulness practitioners often report an enhanced sense of optimism and increased positive emotions, creating a favorable mental environment for overall well-being.

5. **Promotes Better Stress Management:** Mindfulness enables us to perceive stressors more objectively, reducing the intensity of our stress response. Over time, this can lead to a more balanced and calm approach to life's challenges.

Cultivating a Mindful Lifestyle

The beauty of mindfulness is that it doesn't require hours of meditation. It can be practiced anytime, anywhere. Whether you're washing dishes, taking a walk, or simply breathing, each moment offers an opportunity for mindfulness. The key is intentionality and practice.

Overcoming Barriers to Mindfulness

Despite its benefits, practicing mindfulness can be challenging. The modern world is rife with distractions, and our minds often resist quiet contemplation. However, like any skill, mindfulness becomes easier with consistent practice. Start small, perhaps with just five minutes daily, and gradually increase as you become more comfortable.

Supporting Research and Science

It's worth noting that the benefits of mindfulness are not just anecdotal. Numerous scientific studies employing MRI scans and other tools have validated the positive impacts of mindfulness on physical and mental health. This fusion of ancient wisdom with modern science solidifies mindfulness's role in holistic well-being.

Once viewed as a mystical or esoteric practice, mindfulness has secured its place in modern health and wellness discourse. Its benefits, both tangible and intangible, are vast. From improved physical markers of fitness to an elevated state of mental well-being, mindfulness is more than a practice; it's a way of life. By embracing mindfulness, we're improving our health and fostering a more compassionate, attentive, and harmonious world.

Techniques for Incorporating Mindfulness into Daily Life

In our fast-paced, technology-driven world, moments of actual presence can feel like a rarity. With its ancient roots and contemporary relevance, mindfulness offers an antidote to this ceaseless hustle. While the term might evoke images of extended meditation retreats or hours of silent reflection, the essence of mindfulness is surprisingly simple. It can be seamlessly incorporated into our everyday lives. Here's a guide to integrating mindfulness techniques into your daily routine.

1. Begin with Breath

Breathing is the most fundamental act of living. By focusing on it, we root ourselves in the present.

Technique: Take a few moments to notice your breath throughout the day simply. Deeply inhale, hold for a second, then slowly exhale. Pay attention to your chest or abdomen rising and falling or the sensation of the breath entering and exiting your nostrils.

2. Mindful Eating

Turn meals into meditation. Instead of eating on autopilot, savor every bite.

Technique: Observe your food's colors, textures, and aromas. As you eat, note the taste and texture. Chew slowly, appreciating every flavor. This not only enhances your enjoyment of food but also aids digestion.

3. Present Walking

Walking is routine, but how often are we genuinely present

during it?

Technique: As you walk, whether during a morning jog or just moving from one room to another, feel the ground beneath your feet, notice the movement of your legs, and the sensation of air on your skin. This transforms a simple act into a moment of connection with your environment.

4. Mindful Listening

Truly listening, without planning a response or getting lost in our thoughts, is a form of mindfulness.

Technique: When someone is speaking to you, focus entirely on their words. Observe the tone, the emotions behind the terms, and the pauses between them. By being an active listener, you foster better connections with others.

5. Body Scan Meditation

Our bodies constantly send us signals. Tuning into them can ground us in the present.

Technique: Start at the top of your head and move down to your toes. Notice any sensations, tensions, or discomforts in each body part. This practice not only promotes mindfulness but also helps in releasing physical tension.

6. Mindful Tasks

Turn mundane activities into moments of mindfulness.

Technique: Whether washing dishes, brushing your teeth or typing an email, be fully present in the activity. For instance, feel the water's temperature and the sensation of soap on your hands while washing dishes. Such moments can transform routine tasks into mindful breaks.

7. Digital Detox

Our devices can scatter our attention. Setting them aside for a while aids mindfulness.

Technique: Designate specific times in the day when you'll be device-free. Use this time to engage in other mindful activities or observe your surroundings and thoughts.

8. Gratitude Journaling

Gratitude fosters positive mindfulness.

Technique: Jot down three things you're grateful for each day. They can be significant events or simple joys. Over time, this practice will heighten your awareness of joyous moments.

9. Mindful Affirmations

Positive affirmations can anchor us in a positive state of mind.

Technique: Choose a set of positive statements that resonate with you. Every morning or evening, repeat them to yourself, focusing on each word's meaning.

10. Guided Mindfulness Meditation

Guided sessions can be a gateway into more profound mindfulness practices.

Technique: Use apps or online platforms that offer guided sessions. These combine visualization, body scanning, and breathwork to deepen your mindfulness experience.

11. Setting Mindful Alarms

Incorporate mindfulness prompts into your day.

Technique: Set alarms or reminders on your phone with labels like "Take a deep breath" or "What can you hear right now?" These prompts bring you back to the moment.

12. Mindful Decluttering

The state of our surroundings often reflects our inner world.

Technique: Regularly declutter and organize your living space. As you do so, be present in the act. This not only physically clears your environment but also creates mental clarity.

Mindfulness is about cultivating awareness. It's an acknowledgment that every moment is an opportunity to be truly alive. By weaving these techniques into the tapestry of our daily lives, we move from mindless autopilot to a richer, more connected life experience. Remember, mindfulness is not about perfection but practice. Embrace it as a journey, not a destination, and watch as the quality of your everyday moments transforms.

Cultivating Present-Moment Awareness for Enhanced Well-being

Being present and genuinely inhabiting the here and now is more than just a passing trend or a buzzword in wellness circles. It's a foundational mental, emotional, and even physical well-being principle. However, being attuned to the present moment can seem like an uphill task in a world overrun with distractions. Yet, the benefits of such awareness are profound. Let's explore how to cultivate this awareness and its transformative effects on our well-being.

Understanding Present-Moment Awareness

At its core, present-moment awareness is our conscious, active attention to our current experiences, sensations, and thoughts. It's the antithesis of being on "autopilot." It's about noticing, not judging, experiencing, not interpreting.

Why is Present-Moment Awareness Essential?

1. **Reduces Stress:** By focusing on the now, we prevent our minds from dwelling on past regrets or future anxieties. This reduction in rumination can lead to decreased stress levels.

2. **Enhances Emotional Regulation:** Awareness of our present emotions without judgment allows for better emotional clarity, aiding in more effective regulation of our reactions.

3. **Improves Focus and Productivity:** A mind trained to stay in the present can better concentrate on tasks, boosting efficiency and output.

4. **Deepens Relationships:** Being fully present ensures

genuine communication and connection.

5. **Fosters Appreciation:** When we are in the moment, we notice and appreciate the small joys and beauty around us.

How to Cultivate Present-Moment Awareness

1. **Mindful Meditation:** Begin with an essential meditation practice.

Set aside time each day to sit quietly, concentrate on your breathing, and gently refocus your attention anytime it wanders. This straightforward practice strengthens your capacity to be present.

2. **Engage Your Senses:** Make it a habit to check in with your five senses regularly. What do you hear? Smell? Feel? See? Taste? This grounds you and can be done anywhere, from waiting in line to walking.

3. **Single-Tasking:** While multitasking might seem efficient, it often leads to divided attention. Instead, try single-tasking. Dedicate your full attention to one task at a time.

4. **Digital Breaks:** Allocate specific times when you

disconnect from digital devices during the day. This practice reduces the constant influx of information and allows you to be more present.

5. **Nature Immersion:** Spend time outdoors. Nature brings us back to the present, whether feeling the wind, hearing the rustling leaves, or watching a sunset.

6. **Mindful Reminders:** Use Post-it notes, alarms, or even apps that remind you to take a moment, breathe, and be present.

7. **Journaling:** Keeping a daily journal where you note your feelings, sensations, and thoughts can enhance self-awareness and keep you grounded in the present.

8. **Active Listening:** When in a conversation, practice active listening. This means fully concentrating on what is being said, understanding, and responding while being mindful of the emotions and thoughts it evokes.

9. **Yoga:** The practice of yoga isn't just physical. The poses, breathwork, and the philosophy behind it all anchor practitioners in the present moment.

10. **Limit Over-scheduling:** Overloading your schedule can lead to constant forward-thinking and stress. Keep

some unscheduled times in your day for spontaneity and relaxation.

Cultivating present-moment awareness isn't about neglecting the past or ignoring the future. It's about giving the present its due, understanding that it is the only moment where life is truly lived. By embedding the practices mentioned above into your daily life, you will enhance your well-being and experience life with a richness and depth that perhaps you never knew was possible. The present moment, after all, is a gift. Embracing it is our pathway to a fuller, more enriched existence.

CHAPTER 19

THE ROLE OF TECHNOLOGY IN MODERN WELL-BEING

In recent years, there's been a profound shift in how we live, work, and play, primarily driven by technological advances. Technology is interwoven into nearly every facet of cell phones; wearable technology, innovative home products, and virtual reality all play a part in our everyday life. While these advancements have ushered in an era of unprecedented connectivity and convenience, they have also brought forth concerns about their impact on our well-being.

To understand the multifaceted influence of technology on well-being, it's crucial to consider both the positive and negative implications.

The Positive Impacts

Firstly, let's appreciate the advantages. The rise of telemedicine, for instance, has allowed people in remote areas to consult with medical professionals without traveling long distances. This accessibility can be life-changing, particularly for those with limited mobility or resources.

Online platforms, too, have revolutionized the way we communicate. Families separated by continents can now video call and feel a semblance of closeness, which was unimaginable a few decades ago. Similarly, when used mindfully, social media can foster connections, allowing users to find communities that share their interests and experiences.

Moreover, technology has been instrumental in democratizing education. With countless online courses and resources, anyone with an internet connection can learn, ranging from basic literacy to advanced technical skills. This has undoubtedly paved the way for personal and professional growth for many.

The Adverse Impacts

However, this digital revolution has its downsides. An obvious concern revolves around screen time. Prolonged exposure can lead to physical health issues like eye strain, sleep disturbances, and a sedentary lifestyle. There's also the phenomenon known as "text neck," which is the strain on the neck muscles caused by frequently looking down at devices.

On the mental well-being front, the effects can be even

more pronounced. Cognitive overload can result from the continual inundation of information, making concentrating or controlling tension difficult. Comparing ourselves to others on social media platforms, where life often looks picture-perfect, can erode self-worth and exacerbate feelings of inadequacy.

Moreover, the boundary between work and personal life has become increasingly blurred, with emails and work notifications pouring in at all hours. This "always-on" culture can contribute to burnout and hinder relaxation and healing.

Striking a Balance

So, where does this leave us? It's clear that while technology has brought about conveniences and opened up a world of possibilities, it also challenges our physical and mental well-being.

The way forward is to accept technology and engage with it mindfully. This might mean setting clear boundaries, like designating screen-free hours before bedtime or using apps that track and limit usage. It could also involve deliberately creating tech-free zones or times in homes focusing on face-to-face interactions.

Regular digital detoxes, where one disconnects from devices for extended periods, can also rejuvenate. This provides a break from the constant notifications and the pull of the online world, allowing for reflection and a deeper connection with the immediate surroundings.

Balancing Digital Engagement for Improved Physical and Mental Health

In today's digital age, screens dominate much of our time. Our daily activities are interlaced with technology, from professional duties to personal pursuits. While this digital engagement offers convenience and a world of information at our fingertips, it can also impact our physical and mental health. Balancing this engagement becomes pivotal, ensuring we derive the benefits without compromising our well-being.

The Era of Screen Dominance

With the dawn of smartphones, tablets, smartwatches, and other wearable tech, screens are always within arm's reach. Remote work, virtual meetings, and online socializing have intensified our screen time. In addition, streaming platforms, gaming, and social media provide endless entertainment, making it easier to stay glued to screens.

Physical Ramifications of Excessive Screen Time

Over-reliance on screens can manifest in various physical health issues:

1. **Eye Strain:** Prolonged screen use can lead to digital eye strain, characterized by dry eyes, blurred vision, and headaches. This phenomenon, often called Computer Vision Syndrome, arises from staring at screens for extended periods without breaks.

2. **Postural Issues:** Hours spent in front of computers, especially with improper ergonomics, can result in back and neck pain. The ubiquitous use of mobile devices further accentuates the problem, leading to the aptly named "text neck."

3. **Sedentary Lifestyle:** Screen activities are predominantly sedentary. Over time, this lack of movement can contribute to health issues related to obesity, cardiovascular illnesses, and other conditions.

Mental Health Implications

Beyond the physical, the digital world significantly influences our mental landscape:

1.   **Information Overload:** With constant notifications, news cycles, and social media updates, the brain struggles to process the influx, leading to cognitive fatigue.

2.   **Social Media Comparisons:** Platforms portraying idealized versions of reality can spur feelings of inadequacy, jealousy, and lowered self-esteem.

3.   **Sleep Disruptions:** Overexposure to blue light emitted by screens, especially before bedtime, can interfere with the body's melatonin production, hampering sleep quality.

Finding the Digital Balance

Achieving equilibrium between our digital and real-world engagements isn't about shunning technology but about using it judiciously:

1.   **20-20-20 Rule:** To combat eye strain, Take a 20-second break every 20 minutes to concentrate on something 20 feet away. This simple routine can significantly reduce the risks associated with prolonged screen use.

2.   **Ergonomic Setups:** Investing in ergonomic furniture and ensuring the screen is at eye level can prevent postural problems. Additionally, taking regular stretch breaks can combat physical stagnation.

3.   **Digital Detox:** Allocate specific times during the day or week when you intentionally disconnect. This break from screens allows the mind to reset and encourages more tactile, real-world engagements.

4.   **Mindful Consumption:** Instead of mindlessly scrolling through feeds, be selective about your digital consumption. Engage in quality content, limit harmful or provocative material exposure, and curate your online spaces to reflect positivity.

5.   **Tech-Free Bedrooms:** Make the bedroom a tech-free zone to improve sleep or reduce screen engagement an hour before sleeping.

6.   **Physical Activities:** Counterbalance the passive nature of screen activities by incorporating regular physical exercises into your routine. Even straightforward acts like walking significantly alter the situation.

7.   **Quality over Quantity:** Instead of spending hours with fragmented attention, allocate specific durations for focused digital activities. For example, designate time for emails, social media, and entertainment separately. This not only reduces screen time but also enhances productivity.

Finding the right balance is crucial in an age where digital engagement is almost inescapable. By being proactive and setting boundaries, it's possible to coexist with technology in a manner that benefits our physical and mental health. It's not about rejecting the digital realm but harmonizing it with our inherent human needs. By doing so, we safeguard our well-being and enhance the quality of our digital interactions.

Leveraging Technology for Fitness, Mental Health, and Social Interaction

The evolution of technology has brought about a variety of programs and websites created to improve several facets of our life. Technology provides creative answers to age-old problems, from fitness monitors that keep track of our physical activity to applications that let us interact with therapists worldwide. When used judiciously, it can serve as a catalyst in promoting overall well-being, particularly in fitness, mental health, and social interaction.

Fitness: Staying Active in the Digital Age

Wearable Tech: Devices like Fitbit, Garmin, and Apple Watch have revolutionized how we approach fitness. These wearables track our steps, heart rate, sleep patterns, and more, providing detailed insights into our daily activity.

Such real-time feedback can motivate users to move more and achieve their fitness goals.

Virtual Workouts: Online platforms such as Peloton, Zwift, or YouTube fitness channels offer many workout options. Whether it's yoga, HIIT, or dance, users can find a routine that suits them and practice it from home.

Diet and Nutrition Apps: Apps like MyFitnessPal or Cronometer allow users to log their meals, monitor their calorie intake, and ensure they meet their nutritional needs. Such apps often come with extensive food databases, making it easier for users to make informed dietary choices.

Mental Health

Online Therapy: Platforms like BetterHelp and Talkspace connect users with licensed therapists. These services offer flexibility, allowing individuals to seek help per their schedules. For many, the anonymity and convenience of online counseling can make it a more appealing option than traditional therapy.

Meditation and Mindfulness Apps: Headspace, Calm, and Insight Timer are just a few apps designed to guide users through meditation practices. These apps often feature guided sessions, sleep stories, and mindfulness training that can lower anxiety and stress.

Mental Health Trackers: Apps such as Daylio or Moodpath enable users to track their mood and emotional patterns. By reflecting on these patterns, individuals can identify triggers or trends in their mental health, aiding in self-awareness and proactive care.

Social Interaction

Platforms like Facebook, Instagram, and Twitter are examples of social media. While often criticized for various reasons, it also provides avenues for connection. They offer spaces where users can join groups of like-minded individuals, share their experiences, and stay connected with friends and family.

Video Calling Platforms: Tools like Zoom, Skype, and Google Meet have not only facilitated remote work but have also been instrumental in keeping loved ones connected, especially during times when physical meetings were challenging.

Online Communities: Websites like Reddit or Discord host communities centered around countless interests and hobbies. These spaces offer individuals opportunities to connect with others who share their passions, fostering a sense of belonging and camaraderie.

While it's essential to approach technology with a discerning eye, recognizing its potential pitfalls, it's equally crucial to acknowledge the myriad ways it enhances our lives. By leveraging these digital tools mindfully, we can usher in an era where technology truly serves our holistic well-being, bridging the gaps between our physical, mental, and social spheres. In an interconnected world, the key lies in using technology as a bridge to better health and deeper connections, turning the digital landscape into a canvas of possibilities for personal growth.

Techniques for Keeping a Positive Relationship with Technology

In today's hyper-connected era, it's easy to become overwhelmed by the constant barrage of notifications, the endless scroll of social media, and the lure of digital entertainment. While technology offers unparalleled convenience and connection, it also poses potential threats to our mental well-being, physical health, and genuine human interactions. Navigating the digital realm mindfully can ensure that we harness its benefits without succumbing to its pitfalls. Here are strategies to foster a balanced and healthy relationship with technology.

1. Digital Detox Days: Designate certain days or hours when you completely unplug. It could be a full day each week or a few hours each evening. This pause allows you to reconnect with the world around you, fosters mindfulness, and reminds you that there's life beyond the screen.

2. Set Boundaries: Clearly define when and where you use technology. For example, refrain from checking your phone during meals, or establish tech-free zones in the home, such as the bedroom. This can improve sleep quality and enhance the quality of your relationships.

3. Be Selective with Notifications: Turn off non-essential notifications. By only being alerted to crucial messages or updates, you reduce the constant digital interruptions that can scatter your focus.

4. Use Technology Mindfully: Before you pick up your phone or log onto your computer, ask yourself: What is my intention? By being clear about what you hope to achieve, you reduce the chances of getting sucked into the digital vortex of mindless browsing.

5. Embrace Single-Tasking: Contrary to popular belief, multitasking can reduce productivity and increase stress. Focus on one task at a time: reading an article, replying to an email, or watching a video.

6. Prioritize Face-to-Face Interactions: While digital communications are convenient, they should differ from genuine human interaction. Prioritize face-to-face conversations and activities with loved ones, recognizing the depth and richness they bring to relationships.

7. Regularly Review Your Digital Consumption: Every month, take a moment to review the apps and platforms you frequently use. Ask yourself whether they add value to your life or consume your time. Delete or reduce the use of those that don't enhance your well-being.

8. Educate Yourself: Understand the potential downsides of excessive tech use, including digital eye strain, disrupted sleep, and the mental health implications of social media comparison. Being informed can motivate healthier habits.

9. Utilize Tech Tools: Embrace apps or settings that promote well-being. Features like "Do Not Disturb" modes, screen time trackers, or apps that promote relaxation and mindfulness can be beneficial.

10. Physical Health Checks: Ensure you're maintaining good posture, taking breaks to stretch, and observing the formula 20-20-20 (every 20 minutes, To lessen eye strain, gaze somewhere 20 feet away for 20 seconds.

11. Engage in Offline Hobbies: Rediscover or develop offline hobbies – reading, painting, gardening, or any other activity. This provides a break from screens and enhances creativity and cognitive function.

12. Be a Role Model: For parents, it's essential to model healthy technology use for their children. Demonstrating a balanced approach instills these values in the next generation.

Maintaining a healthy relationship with technology is akin to any other relationship in our lives – it requires effort, understanding, and periodic reassessment. In an era defined by digital connection, achieving this balance ensures that technology remains a tool for enhancement, not an impediment to our overall well-being.

CHAPTER 20

CONCLUSION

The Four Spheres of Well Being

A conceptual framework known as the "four spheres of health and wellness" helps people better comprehend how the mind- body relationship functions. They are also physical, spiritual, psychological, and emotional. We can experience illness in the mind and body when there is stagnation in one or more of the four spheres. We experience health and wellness when all four spheres are in motion. Therefore, if you are experiencing any discomfort, try asking yourself these questions:

- Where do I feel stranded in the four spheres?

- On a scale of 1 to 10, how stressed am I, and where in my body am I feeling it?

- Which tool in my toolbox would be most useful right now?

Emotional Sphere: Our four main emotions are listed in the emotional sphere (happy, sad, anger, and fear). We go through these emotions in all their shapes and intensity levels throughout the day. If we let them, emotions are fluid, meaning they change over time like ocean waves. Depending on how we think, some emotions linger longer than others. We can find our flow in this area if we learn to be conscious of our emotions in relation to our thoughts.

Psychological Sphere: According to neuroscientists, we have more than 80,000 thoughts and feelings each day. And guess what? Not all of them are original to us. We often receive messages like "I'm not smart enough to...," and "I'll never be able to accomplish..." from people like our parents or other major caregivers, friends, and teachers. I lack the courage to. Knowing that our thoughts are real yet may not be true is beneficial. Our thoughts shape our views, therefore if we can distinguish between what is true and what is false, we can succeed in this area.

Try asking yourself the following questions and recording your answers if you want to become more conscious of your thoughts:

- Are these ideas real or imaginary?

- What are the narratives and notions I hold about myself?

Spiritual Sphere: How do you relate to other people? to a Superior Being? to the cosmos? The prefrontal cortex, the newest section of the brain, is the entrance to your best self. By using this area of the brain, we can build neuronal connections with the amygdala, the region of the brain that controls the fight-or-flight response. This connection makes things simple in this area. We connect with our spiritual selves and our energy systems when we do so. This can be accomplished through a variety of practices, such as mindfulness, prayer, music, and art.

Physical Sphere: Our bodies are intangible. We might easily become so preoccupied with the physical selves that we forget about our other realms, or we can get so engrossed in our thoughts and emotions that we find it difficult to be in our bodies. Deep breathing exercises are the easiest approach to reunite your mind and body: Breath in for four counts, hold for four counts, and then exhale for six counts through your lips. You will feel even more grounded if you combine a mantra (suchI let go and go with the flow) with the essential oil of your choosing. What's my body telling me? is another question you may try asking yourself.

These Dimensions are Interconnected

People frequently associate wellness with physical health — including diet, exercise, and weight control — but it encompasses so much more. Integrating physical, mental, and spiritual well-being, wellness nourishes the body, stimulates the mind, and uplifts the spirit. It is a lifestyle and tailored approach to living life in a way that "allows you to become the best kind of person that your potentials, circumstances, and fate will enable" even if it always includes working toward health.

For our own sake as much as the sake of the people we care about and who care about us, wellness demands strong self-stewardship. Wellness is both a professional and a personal obligation for those working in the helping industries, like those of us in veterinary medicine. We have an ethical responsibility to take care of our own health and well-being in order to provide patients and clients with high-quality services. According to the Green Cross Standards of Self Care Guidelines, no scenario or person can excuse abandoning it. Sufficient self-care keeps us from hurting others we serve.

Physical, intellectual, emotional, social, spiritual, vocational, financial, and environmental wellness are 8 interrelated dimensions. All of the dimensions must be taken into consideration since, over time, ignoring one will have a negative impact on the others and, eventually, on one's health, well-being, and quality of life. However, they do not need to be evenly balanced. Instead, we ought to aspire for the "personal harmony" that seems most true to us. Naturally, every one of us has different goals, strategies, and objectives, as well as different ideas about what it means to live a full life.

It might be difficult to choose the best course of action for your health and well-being. Although we are aware of what is best for us and how we might improve, we may choose not to do so or, if we do, we may eventually revert to our old habits. Many things affect human behavior, including what we do, how we do it, and whether we are successful. Two of these things, self- regulation, and habits, are particularly important when it comes to wellness.

Self-regulation

Effective human functioning is largely dependent on self-regulation. It is "our capacity to direct our conduct and control our impulses in order to satisfy certain requirements, accomplish particular objectives, or realize particular ideals." It enables us to make decisions that are in line with our core principles and our long- and short-term best interests. There is only one drawback: since self-regulation demands mental energy, the brain is constantly looking for methods to save it.

Habits

Contrarily, habits use up very little energy. "Any behavior that can be reduced to a routine is one less behavior that we must spend time and energy consciously thinking about and deciding upon," writes Duhigg, author of The Power of Habit: Why We Do What We Do in Life and Business. With the cognitive economy and performance efficiency of habits, the brain can save self-control power to concentrate on life's big decisions and free us to do intelligent things like think back on the past and make plans for the future.

Habits have great power. Habits determine our basic existence and, eventually, our future because they account for around 40% of our repetitive daily activity. In actuality, the key to wellness is habits. Habits have a significant impact on one's health, well-being, and quality of life, for better or worse. If you want to enhance things, you should consider your habits since if you alter your behaviors for the better; your life will also improve.

A habit is defined as "an action that is repeated, cued by a particular environment, frequently occurs without much awareness or conscious intent, and is learned by frequent repetition" in the technical sense. The phrase "When I see a cue, I will complete a routine in order to obtain a reward" can be thought of as a formula that the brain automatically follows. According to studies, habits are encoded in brain structures once they are created and can only be strengthened by forming new, stronger habits. They are extremely challenging to alter because of this. It involves rewiring the brain, not merely using willpower (i.e., self-control). You must establish new routines in order to break a habit: Maintain the previous cue and give the old reward while incorporating a new routine.

It's challenging to introduce new routines. Despite our best efforts and knowledge of what is healthy for us, habits often force us to continue acting in the same way. Any of us may attest to the fact that they are challenging to alter. But by focusing on two key components—self-awareness and strategies—we can increase our chances of success. Both are necessary for effective habit formation.

Self-awareness

If you pay attention to who you are and incorporate routines that capitalize on your talents, tendencies, and strengths, change becomes much more attainable. You can develop the habits that work for you by being self-aware. Think about variations in circadian rhythms, for instance. Our circadian rhythms, which reflect our innate tendencies for sleep and waking, have an impact on our energy and productivity throughout the day. If, for instance, you choose to wake up an hour earlier each day to exercise when you happen to be a "night owl" rather than a "morning lark," your chances of success in improving your fitness won't increase.

Self-awareness involves understanding of one's other characteristics, such as whether one is a sprinter, procrastinator, under- or over-buyer, lover of abundance or simplicity, finisher or opener, and fan of familiarity or novelty. You should also consider whether you prefer taking tiny or large measures and whether your focus is on promotion or prevention.

Strategies

If you select tactics that increase your chances of success, change also becomes more attainable. These techniques include scheduling, investing in accountability systems, abstaining, adjusting convenience levels, planning safeguards, spotting justifications and erroneous assumptions, using distractions,rewards, and treats, pairing activities, and starting with routinesthat bolster self-control. Because it takes 66 days for new habits to take root, the more tactics that are utilized to develop a single new behavior will have the greatest chance of success.

Change your behavior to improve your life.

Change might take a very long time. Repeated failures and experimentation are sometimes necessary. However, the effortsare undeniably valuable for continued improvement, and one achievement frequently leads to another. Are you going toaccept yourself or expect more from yourself when it comes to habits, wellness, and the health, well-being, and quality of life that you desire? "Are you going to care about yourself ordisregard yourself?" and "Are you going to appreciate the moment or consider the future?"

A dynamic, ever-evolving, shifting process, wellness. It is a way of life, a tailored approach to living that enables you to develop into the most positive version of yourself that your capabilities, environment, and destiny will permit. The decisions you make today will determine your present and future; the past is history. Don't stress about doing things perfectly; just start, and develop into the greatest person you can be.

What is a Good Life?

Every person hopes to lead a good life. The issue is that we all have varying definitions of what a "happy life" entails. Some people aspire to live a life of integrity, contentment, and joy. Others aim to achieve wealth, social prestige, and fame in the belief that these qualities will enable them to live fulfilling lives. In fact, they immediately link having money and material possessions to living a pleasant life.

Some people entirely neglect other people's needs in their pursuit of a good life, while others see assisting others as a way to live a good life. Who gets to choose what makes a good life still remains an open subject.

Not everyone who appears to be living "the dream" or "the good life" actually is. Consider the notorious Colombian drug lord Pablo Escobar as an example. Yes, he lived comfortably. Escobar, after all, is known to have been the richest criminal in history. He owned opulent homes, race vehicles, and private jets. And I have no doubt that he finds joy and fulfillment in his life. Was his life, however, a happy one? Definitely not.

As you can see, there may be a significant distinction between leading a good life and leading the good life. Not everyone who is happy with their life is also happy with their life.

The phrase "the good life" describes a (desirable) condition that is largely characterized by a high standard of living or by abiding by moral and ethical principles. Living the good life can be expressed in one of two ways: either by an extravagant lifestyle replete with material possessions, or by making an effort to live in line with the moral, legal, and religious laws of one's nation or culture. As a result, the term can be used to refer to both the pursuit of wealth, material goods, or luxury as well as the endeavor to live a worthwhile, sincere, and meaningful life.

What really constitutes the good life and what makes it possible?

Almost all of us have preconceived notions about what it means to live the good life. Some people define the good life as having unlimited access to food and drink while watching television or playing video games. Others believe that living well involves spending time outdoors contemplating and philosophizing about life. Some people only want to make the most of their time by doing good and useful things, like working to improve the world. Others consider pleasure, prosperity, and achieving all of their (material) desires to be essential elements of the ideal life.

These instances bring up a significant point. Some people define the good life as a life spent continually pursuing their objectives through menial tasks. Others see it as the pursuit of individual achievement and the desire to make a positive impacton the world.

These instances bring up a significant point. Some people define the good life as a life spent continually pursuing their objectives through menial tasks. Others see it as the pursuit of individual achievement and the desire to make a positive impacton the world.

The next thing we need to consider is whether a high quality of living alone might truly define the good life. If this were the case, then pursuing one's desires and monetary goals would constitute the majority of living the good life. Human aspirations can be limitless, but the earth's resources are relatively finite, as we all know. Therefore, the (over)excellent life of one set of people may prohibit others from living the "high-standard-of- living good life" or it may prevent future generations from ever living the good life.

A high level of living is undoubtedly a component of the good life. However, money and prosperity do not, by themselves, constitute the good life. As a result, it would be severely constrained and unbalanced.

In support of this argument, the well-known philosophers Socrates and Plato characterize the good life as essentially involving self-mastery, self-examination, and community service. They believed that self-control and civic responsibility were integral parts of having a decent life. As a result, achieving self-mastery and making a positive impact on your community were essential components of a happy life.

Benefits of Living and Eating Clean

You've probably heard of clean eating if you're attempting to eat healthily. But what does it really include, and what foods are appropriate for a clean eating diet? In essence, it is choosing whole foods in their unprocessed, natural forms over items that have been heavily processed and have additional sugars, chemicals, and preservatives.

The specifics depend on how stringent you are, however, the fundamental principles of clean eating are straightforward and include things like:

- Produce and fruits

- Fermented foods like kimchi and sauerkraut

- Whole legumes and beans (soaked, drained, and cooked)

- Miso, tofu, and natto are examples of soy products.

- Nuts and seeds, especially unroasted or unsalted varieties

- Whole grains including quinoa, brown rice,

barley, and oats. both faro

- Olive oil, avocado oil, coconut oil, and walnutoils are examples of cold-pressed culinary oils.

- fresh poultry and meat
- organic eggs and dairy (in moderation)
- spices and herbs
- Drink plenty of water

Of course, not all processed food is unhealthy. As an illustration, pasteurization renders dairy products safe for humanconsumption. Similar to fermentation, freezing some foods can prolong or improve their nutritional value.

What advantages do clean eating offer?

When you follow a clean eating regimen, you are more likelyto consume a balanced meal that is mostly composed of fruits, vegetables, and whole grains, which give your body healthy fuel and long-lasting energy. Additionally, it advises you to avoid foods that have fillers and toxic components that your body mustfilter out.

High water content and balanced mineral and vitamin levels can be found in clean diet meals. These foods can enhance bodily performance generally and keep the body in homeostasis,or perfect balance:

- Weight loss: Because they often contain fewer calories than junk food, it is simpler to keep a caloric deficit.

- Mood: Rich in minerals and antioxidants that improve mood and general mental health.

- Gut health: Antioxidants and fiber-rich foods promote the development of good gut bacteria.

- Immune system: Foods high in minerals and antioxidants can support a healthy immune system.

- Aids in the prevention of chronic illnesses like cancer and cardiovascular disease.

- Anti-aging: Prevents oxidative stress from accelerating aging.

- Anti-inflammatory: Can lessen long-term inflammation, which is linked to the emergence of serious chronic conditions.

How to maintain healthy eatingpractices?

It can be challenging to maintain a clean eating regimen, especially for beginners. Since bad eating habits and a sedentary lifestyle frequently coexist, it's extra harder if you don't follow aregular exercise routine.

But if you start off gently, you might succeed. You may giveup if there are too many limits placed on you or if you find it difficult to follow a new food plan. So, make an effort to maintain flexibility, and keep in mind that even if you falter along the road, what matters is that you remain focused on yourlong-term goals for nutritious eating. Clean eating will become easier to include in your lifestyle with time.

How to Improve Your Well-Being?

Take a break from your robotic routine and choose healthy behaviors if you are someone who is constantly preoccupied with work and other things while paying little attention to your health and well-being.

A psychologist claims that eating healthily and exercising will instantly help your body and brain manage stress, despair, and anxiety. Balance, continuous improvement, and acceptanceare the keys to true well-being.

Here are some tried-and-true strategies to assist you to enhance your wellbeing:

- **Get enough rest**

It could seem like the most obvious advice, but believe me when I say that the majority of people don't adhere to the fundamental steps for their general welfare. Our bodies require adequate sleep and rest in order to recover and refuel with energy. For daily physical and mental activities, this healing is crucial.

The hormones that are directly linked to our emotions and mood are controlled by getting enough sleep. Most frequently, when you experience emotional instability or irritability, the likelihood that your body is not getting enough sleep is high. Nearly 6 to 7 hours of sleep per day are required for an adult body. Therefore, be sure to get enough rest.

- **Consume a Healthy Diet**

You won't get the benefits you need from sleep on its own. To ensure that your body gets enough nutrients, you need to consume a healthy, balanced diet. How healthy your inside system is determined by the stuff you eat. Additionally, it aids in identifying your emotional well-being and any mental diseases like depression.

Your body will suffer major health issues if it is deficient in key nutrients. You also experience emotional distress and anxiety. According to health and wellness professionals, you should consume enough fruits and vegetables. Additionally, consuming lentils and nuts helps to strengthen your heart. As much as you can, try to stay away from coffee, sugar, and processed foods.

- **Put Your Body in the Sun**

Seasonal Affective Disorder, sometimes known as SAD, is caused by a vitamin D deficiency. Endorphins—also known as "happy hormones"—that are responsible for the brain's productivity are released when you are exposed to sunlight.

Take a break from your routine and spend some time outside in the sun. However, wear sunscreen to avoid getting burned.

- **Managing Stress**

Although it can be challenging to avoid stress these days, there are ways to deal with it. It is crucial to have good coping mechanisms for stress. Try to stay away from stressful circumstances to achieve that. If your stress is out of control, write down the reasons why as well as any steps you may take to alter your behavior, mood, or even circumstance.

- **Exercise Daily:**

Your body's blood flow improves when you stay physically active and work out every day. You feel more energized, awake, and cognitively alert as a result of the increased blood flow andoxygenation.

If you work in an office, exercises and physical activities are more crucial. Exercise keeps your mind in good condition in addition to keeping your body in shape. For that, you don't needto join an expensive gym. A short stroll with your pet or a dailymorning stroll suffices. The key is to establish it as a daily routine.

Exercise not only improves your mental health but also yourbones and muscles, protecting you against various types of accidents when exercising or performing your regular chores.

- **Stay away from alcohol and smoking.**

No matter how much money you spend on your health or how hard you try, if you continue to drink and smoke, your efforts will be in vain.

To live a healthy life, give up drinking and smoking.

- **As much as you can, be social.**

The two main causes of depression and other mental and physical diseases are isolation and poor communication. Try to set aside some time for friends and socialize with them, despite how busy your family and professional lives are.

A man needs social interaction to maintain his health. Having conversations with others reduces stress. If you've heard of laughter therapy, you'll know that laughing with others also has the same objective of lowering stress. Everyone desires acceptance and connection, and these needs can only be metthrough social interaction.

- **Discover and engage in new hobbies**

Our hobbies keep us occupied and interested. You take positive efforts to enhance your emotional well-being when you are interested in and like performing certain things. It also relieves your brain of the stress of daily life and work. Developing new interests is a terrific way to improve mental andemotional health.

- **Understand How to Be Present**

The primary cause of mood swings, despair, and anxiety is when a person is still preoccupied with the past. Self-critical thoughts like "why people did this to me" take not just enjoyment but also cause a person to overlook opportunities thatthey now have to give.

Try to avoid dwelling too much on the future and learn to livein the here and now.

Simple advice

Take nothing in life too seriously. People who endeavor to keep themselves happy, smile more, and maintain their happiness have a higher quality of life than people who constantly worry. Children laugh 200 times every day but adultsonly do so 15 times, claims a study.

A quality existence depends on maintaining your happiness and smiling more.

As we reach the culmination of "lifestyle after COVID -19 ", the interconnectedness of physical, mental, emotional, and social well-being becomes clear. In these challenging times marked by a global pandemic, we have grappled with an external threat and internal realizations about health, relationships, and our relationship with the digital world.

The chapters on physical well-being emphasize nourishing our bodies through clean eating, regular exercise, and understanding nutrition at its core. A sound body is foundational, acting as the vessel through which we experience life.

Our exploration into mental and emotional well-being underscored the importance of understanding our psyche, taming negative behaviors, and cultivating a space of self-awareness and self-love. Given the external stressors, taking care of our mental health becomes paramount in these tumultuous times.

The deep dive into social well-being has highlighted the importance of genuine connections, mastering essential social skills, and building healthy relationships. The pandemic emphasized our intrinsic need for connection, making it necessary to strengthen our social bonds and support systems.1

Our engagement with digital platforms has grown exponentially in the age of rapid technological advancements. This book has underscored the need to leverage technology effectively while safeguarding our well-being from potential drawbacks. Establishing a balance, setting boundaries, and using technology as an enabler rather than a dominator emerged as key themes.

The post-COVID world requires a holistic approach to well-being. As we navigate this new landscape, we must remember that each sphere of our well-being is interconnected, influencing and reinforcing the others. A comprehensive, balanced approach, filled with mindfulness, intentionality, and a commitment to continuous learning, will ensure that we survive in this new era and truly thrive. Embrace the journey, for it is through challenges that we discover our resilience, capacity for change, and growth potential.